T0321672

THE FUTURE OF
HOMO

THE FUTURE OF
HOMO

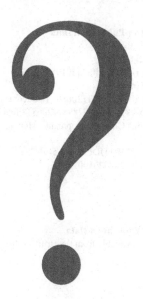

Michel Odent
Primal Health Research Centre, UK

World Scientific

:W JERSEY • LONDON • SINGAPORE • BEIJING • SHANGHAI • HONG KONG • TAIPEI • CHENNAI • TOKYO

Published by

World Scientific Publishing Co. Pte. Ltd.
5 Toh Tuck Link, Singapore 596224
USA office: 27 Warren Street, Suite 401-402, Hackensack, NJ 07601
UK office: 57 Shelton Street, Covent Garden, London WC2H 9HE

Library of Congress Cataloging-in-Publication Data
Names: Odent, Michel, 1930–   author.
Title: The future of Homo / Michel Odent.
Description: Hackensack, NJ : World Scientific, [2019] | Includes
    bibliographical references and index.
Identifiers: LCCN 2019025052 | ISBN 9789811206801 (hardcover) |
    ISBN 9789811207549 (paperback) | ISBN 9789811206818 (ebook)
Subjects: LCSH: Natural childbirth. | Child development. | Human beings--Forecasting. |
    Human evolution--Philosophy.
Classification: LCC RG661 .O343 2019 | DDC 618.4/5--dc23
LC record available at https://lccn.loc.gov/2019025052

British Library Cataloguing-in-Publication Data
A catalogue record for this book is available from the British Library.

For any available supplementary material, please visit
https://www.worldscientific.com/worldscibooks/10.1142/11458#t=suppl

Printed in Singapore

"I dedicate this book
to my unborn great grandchild
and the forthcoming generations".

Contents

Acknowledgments

I am indebted to several individuals who offered their insights while I was raising questions about the future of Homo. I am thinking in particular of the World Scientific publishing editor Sook Cheng Lim, who gave me irreplaceable advice regarding the title of the book and the limits of its contents. I am also grateful to Samantha Price and Liliana Lammers, two "wise women" who shared their experience and perspectives with me on a quasi-daily basis.

Introduction

In the Age of Question Marks

Since our contemporaries constantly have to deal with unprecedented situations, question marks are symbolic of the current phase of the history of life on planet Earth. Throughout this book, we'll analyse radically new situations, before phrasing appropriate questions. As a general rule, we consider it premature to express opinions and theories, and to suggest solutions.

At a time when it is commonplace to debate on the long-term effects of human activities without considering the probable transformations of Homo, we cannot avoid a preliminary question:

How to reach an audience made up of open-minded people who are turned towards the future but have not yet realised that the critical period surrounding birth has been radically transformed during the past decades?

1 The Broken Mirror

Abstract

In the age of cultural blindness related to overspecialisation and information overload, we accumulate reasons to focus on boundaries between perspectives. For example, the concept of "physiological birth preparation", which is outside the dominant perspectives, hardly attracts any attention. We use it to refer to a short period that is not yet established labour, and during which fast physiological changes are taking place. It is easy to emphasise the importance of the topic and to phrase urgent questions at a time when labour induction, pre-labour caesarean section, and many aspects of modern lifestyle are frequent and powerful interferences. This example is the point of departure of a book that should not be classified as medical. One of our objectives is to emphasise that childbirth and specifically human diseases are obligatory topics to explore the nature of Homo. We use interdisciplinary perspectives to raise questions about the future of our species and the limits of human adaptability. We constantly refer to "Homo", because pure Sapiens do not exist: we are all hybrids.

Since the turn of the millennium, the amount of knowledge we all have at our disposal has reached an unexpected order of magnitude. Today, by associating a small number of keywords, everybody has access to countless established facts regarding highly precise topics.

This is also the time when the word "specialist" is usually associated with a positive connotation.

Can "Information Bombardment" Make Us Blind?

At such a turning point in the history of mankind, it is worth recalling that half a millennium ago there were still scholars who were supposed to have acquired an encyclopaedic knowledge. One of the prototypes of such scholars was Pico della Mirandola, from Florence, famous for his 900 theses on a variety of subjects. According to Pascal, he knew "de omni re scibili" (about every knowable thing). In such a context and until recently, "erudition" was associated with a positive connotation.

The time has come to express warnings about the negative effects of "information bombardment". At the very end of the 20th century, I had already described emerging effects of information technology by using the analogy of the broken mirror.[1] It is as if, until recently, we could study human nature through a mirror that was not well polished. The image was fuzzy, details indistinct. But it was still possible to see the unpolished mirror in its entirety. The same mirror suddenly became brilliantly polished, but it is as though it is broken into thousands of pieces. Experts who know so much about a tiny piece of the fragmented mirror are unable to see the way it links with the other pieces that make up the whole.

The Marine Chimpanzee

As an example of a cultural blindness related to overspecialisation, I'll mention the current collective difficulty to consider Homo a primate adapted to coastal areas. For each of the countless particularities of our own genus Homo in the framework of mammal species, even the most mysterious, specialised scientists can offer multiple plausible interpretations in terms of evolutionary advantages and adaptation to different environments. Meanwhile, there is no interest in a possible unifying theoretical framework.[2] However, we have at our disposal such a unifying framework, based on a simple rule: when a trait is mysterious, and apparently specific to humans, we must look at what we have in common with mammals adapted to the sea.

Here are examples of such human traits:

- The huge development of the brain: mammals adapted to the sea generally have higher "encephalisation quotient" than their cousins on land.
- An enzymatic system that is not very effective at making a molecule of fatty acid ("DHA") which is essential to feed the brain. This molecule is abundant and preformed in the sea food chain.
- Iodine is the most common nutritional deficiency among humans, except among those who have access to the sea food chain.
- Nakedness and a layer of fat under the skin are traits shared with sea mammals.
- The skin of human newborn babies is covered with vernix caseosa (literally cheesy varnish)…like the skin of newborn seals.
- Human mothers do not eat the placenta…a common point with sea mammals.
- The sense of smell of human beings is mysteriously weak. It is the same among whales. When they separated from hoofed mammals about 60 million years ago and migrated to water, their sense of smell nearly disappeared.[3]
- Body temperature control through the loss of sweat is not a costly mechanism if we think of the human being as a primate adapted to environments where water and minerals are available without restriction.
- A low larynx, which gives us the ability to breathe through our nose or our mouth, is an anatomical particularity shared with sea lions and dugongs.

- A prominent nose is a feature shared with the proboscis, a primate who lives in coastal wetlands and is an excellent distance swimmer.
- The human vagina, like that of sea mammals, is long and oblique, and is protected by a hymen.
- The human apolipoprotein E gene has more similarities with the one of sea mammals than with the one of land mammals (including common chimpanzees and bonobos).[4] Apolipoprotein E is the principal cholesterol carrier in the brain.
- One of the most common abnormalities (or particularities) among humans is a webbing between the second and the third toe. When a congenital abnormality is an addition, it usually means that the feature was there for a reason during the evolutionary process.
- A narrowing of the thoracic aorta ("coarctation of the aorta") is common among humans and seals.
- Growth of bone (exostosis) in the ear canal is particular to humans who are frequent swimmers, and also whales and seals.[5]
- Menopause, and prolonged life after reproduction, is a feature shared by humans, killer whales and short-finned pilot whales.

If we add recent spectacular advances in population genetics, and what we are learning about fluctuations of sea levels and also about archaic humans as navigators, it appears difficult to avoid considering a radically new vision of man.

Adaptation to "Information Bombardment"

In such a context, adaptation to information overload has become a priority. We urgently need to learn how several ways to channel human curiosity and hunger for information may be combined.

One way is to develop the art of detecting and selecting valuable and potentially useful information: we need to modernise the ancient art of "finding a needle in a haystack". The obligatory first step would be to transcend the current classifications of available data. Many pieces of knowledge remain useless as long as they are not easily found through the usual channels and remain isolated. This is why one of my objectives has been to gather, in a computerised database, the results of studies that are unrelated according to the current classifications.

Since the 1980s, through the Primal Health Research Database ("primalhealthresearch.com"), we bring together epidemiological studies that explore correlations between the "primal period" and what happens later on in life in terms of health and personality traits. The primal period goes from conception until the first birthday. We need to screen a great diversity of scientific and medical journals to occasionally detect one publication that belongs to this framework.

Here is an example of a published piece of information that has remained nearly undetected, in spite of its great scientific value and probable practical implications. According to a Swedish study, the longer the time a boy has spent in the womb, the smaller the risks are of developing a prostate cancer in old age.[6] This study has a great scientific value. The authors looked at an enormous cohort of men born between 1889 and 1941 in Stockholm. Eight hundred and thirty four cases of prostate cancer were identified from the cohort between 1958 and 1994, with 1880 controls included in the study. The reasons why this study has remained ignored are obvious in the current phase of the history of information technology. First, it was published in a serious but highly specialised scientific journal that is not read by health practitioners. Furthermore, even if the published article had reached practitioners, it is highly probable, for obvious reasons, that most readers would not have gone beyond the title: experts in prostate cancer are not interested in foetal life, while obstetricians and midwives are not conditioned to think long term and are not interested in the risks for a newborn boy to develop a prostate cancer one day.

This is why it is urgent to develop new ways to classify scientific data in order to facilitate the detection of established knowledge with practical implications. In the exemplary case of the links between duration of foetal life and risk of prostate cancer, it would be worth considering the practical implications.

In such a context, an objective of this book is to focus on one obligatory way to minimise the current high degree of blindness related to "information bombardment". In the age of overspeciali-sation, we must train ourselves to focus on the continuity between phases of life that are usually looked at in isolation. This will lead us, as a point of departure, to analyse the concept of "physiological birth preparation". It is easy to emphasise the importance of the topic and to phrase urgent questions at a time when this phase of human life is frequently eliminated or shortened through labour induction or pre-labour caesarean section.

To achieve our goal, we'll first recall how important aspects of the birth process among humans may be understood today. Then it will be easy to realise that there are in late pregnancy maternal physiological modifications that prepare the crucial event.

After presenting "physiological birth preparation" as a prototype of the phases of transition that need to be looked at in depth, we'll find opportunities to enlarge the topic and to present the emerging art of creating links between tiny pieces of the fragmented mirror.

Since the concept of preparation is akin to the concept of anticipation, we'll be constantly turned towards the future and we'll offer reasons to urgently enlarge the frameworks of futurology and evolutionary thinking...without prophesying.

Focusing on "the future of Homo" is symbolic of a new way of thinking. More common questions, such as: "Has the human game begun to play itself out?" are related to human activities.[7] When wondering: "What kind of Homo can play itself out?", we suggest that we should first consider probable transformations of our species.

The reason why we do not associate the word Homo with the word sapiens needs to be clarified. Three centuries ago, when Carl Linnaeus formalised the modern way of naming living organisms, he did not bother to define Homo. He had no reason to think that the genus homo would ever have additional members. The only species belonging to the Genus Homo was called "sapiens". This is why, even today, the term Homo has not been properly defined. It may be used with an enlarged sense, referring to all the hominids that separated from the other members of the chimpanzee family (the genus Pan) about six million years ago. It may be used as a synonym of "hominin", including all apes more closely related to humans than chimpanzees. It may also be used with a restricted sense, referring to modern human beings.

Throughout this book, when using the word Homo, we are referring to "great apes", characterised by a huge brain, more precisely those with an adult brain volume that has reached another order of magnitude compared with all other hominins. This framework includes modern humans and other variants of the known or not yet known "big-brained hominins" such as Neanderthal and Denisovan. Today it is becoming difficult to separate these variants of the "big-brained hominins", since we are accumulating data concerning the multiple and diverse lasting effects of interbreeding. We may even claim that Neanderthal and Denisovan have not disappeared, since modern humans from Asian and European origin share with them gene variants that are associated with physiological particularities. Pure Sapiens do not exist. We are hybrids.

References

1. Odent M (1999) *The Scientification of Love*. Free Association Books, London.
2. Odent M (2017) *The Birth of Homo, the Marine Chimpanzee*. Pinter & Martin, London.

3. Kishida T, Thewissen JGM, Hayakawa T, *et al.* (2015) Aquatic adaptation and the evolution of smell and taste in whales. *Zoological Lett* **1**:9. doi.org/10.1186/s40851-014-0002-z.
4. Davis RW, Pierotti VR, Lauer SJ, *et al.* (1991) Lipoproteins in pinnipeds: analysis of a high molecular weight form of apolipoprotein E. *J Lipid Res* **32(6)**:1013–23.
5. Peter Rhys-Evans (2019) The Waterside Ape: An Alternative Account of Human Evolution. CRC Press, Boca Raton.
6. Ekbom A, Wuu J, Adami HO, *et al.* (2000) Duration of gestation and prostate cancer risk in offspring. *Cancer Epidem Biomar* **9(2)**:221–3.
7. Bill McKibben (2019) *Falter: Has the Human Game Begun To Play Itself Out?* Henry Holt, New York City.

The Main Dish and the Sauce

Abstract

Until now, studies of birth physiology among humans were based on interpretations of difficulties. This is why the comparative importance of mechanical factors has been overestimated by theoreticians. We should first interpret the well-known fact that, occasionally, women who are not special from a morphological perspective can give birth easily and quickly, while others need medical intervention after days of hard labour. This enormous discrepancy leads us to understand that birth physiology is first and foremost a chapter of brain physiology. It is essential to realise that the part of the brain that has reached an extremely high level of development in our species — the "new brain" or neocortex — does not always play the role of a tool at the service of vital physiological functions. On the contrary, in some particular situations, it can inhibit and weaken such functions. It is as if the tool may become the master. The main objective of this chapter is to popularise the concept of neocortical inhibition. A reduced self-control, as an effect of a reduced neocortical activity, appears as the main factor that makes human birth possible. When this solution found by nature is understood, it becomes easy to analyse and summarise the basic needs of a labouring woman: she needs to feel protected against all possible neocortical stimulations. The keyword is protection. The main stimulants of neocortical activity are well-known: language, light, and all attention-enhancing situations.

After using the visual analogy of the broken mirror to illustrate one of the effects of information overload and overspecialisation, we might use the analogy of the broken clock, related to the concept of time, as a way to become aware of our lack of interest and curiosity for periods of transition between physiological events.

Changing the Focus

Until now, books, scientific articles and lectures about birth physiology in the particular case of Homo were based on morphological and mechanical considerations. The importance of mechanical factors has been obviously overestimated.

Among humans, the point of departure should not be to interpret the difficulties of childbirth. It should be to interpret the well-known fact that, occasionally, women who are not special from a morphological perspective can give birth easily within some minutes, while others need a caesarean section after days of hard labour. This enormous discrepancy should be the basis of the central question. Valuable recent studies have confirmed the huge diversity in the shape of the human female pelvis.[1] If the evolutionary process has not selected one particular kind of pelvis, it implies that we must reconsider the comparative importance of mechanical factors.

Today we are in a position to understand that birth physiology is first and foremost a chapter of brain physiology and that the key to go a step further in our understanding of human nature is to assimilate and popularise the concept of neocortical inhibition. It is essential to realise that the part of the brain that has reached an extreme development in our species — the "new brain" or neocortex — does not always play the role of a tool at the service of vital physiological functions. On the contrary, in some particular situations, it can inhibit and weaken such functions. It is as if the tool may become the master.

This is why the concept of neocortical inhibition is the "main dish" of most of my books. To make it easier to digest, I present this term with different "sauces". For example, in "Primal Health", published in 1986, I suggested that to understand the concept of "health" we must first smash the barriers between the different parts of the "Primal Adaptive system", namely the nervous system, the immune system, and the hormonal system. This was an opportunity to refer to the relationship between the neocortex and archaic brain structures and to claim that in humans the neocortex is so highly developed that it often tends to overcontrol and repress the activity of the "primal brain" to such an extent that "it inhibits those physiological functions which are most vulnerable, such as childbirth and the sexual act". More than 20 years later, in "The Functions of the Orgasms: the Highways to Transcendence", the concept of reduced neocortical control was presented as crucial to interpret the subjective aspects of the "foetus ejection reflex", "the milk ejection reflex", the "sperm ejection reflex" and, in general, all transcendent emotional states that can give access to another reality than space and time reality. It is significant that in the indexes of my books, the term neocortex (or neocortical inhibition) is usually the most productive one.

To improve our understanding of how a pregnant woman is physiologically preparing herself to give birth, we shall not follow the apparently logical chronological order. We'll go backwards. We'll first unhesitatingly refer again, particularly for newcomers in the field of human reproductive life, to the concept of "neocortical inhibition", which is challenging our cultural conditioning. Furthermore, before focusing on the birth process, we'll make more precise, through anecdotes and scientific data, the significance of this concept.

I have learned from experience about the effects of anecdotes that are easily interpreted. One of them is the case of a couple making love. While they are in a pre-orgasmic state, the woman suddenly asks her partner: "Have you paid the bill for the car insurance?" It is obvious for everybody that being asked a question is a neocortical stimulation that can interfere with physiological processes.

Among scientific studies, those about the sense of smell are particularly useful. All students in human nature have a special interest in olfaction, because it is mysteriously weak in our species, even if there are differences between ethnic groups explained by genetic and cultural factors. We have already mentioned that a weak sense of smell is a trait shared by humans and sea mammals such as whales. A significant study from Israel has convincingly suggested that neo-cortical inhibition is undoubtedly one the main factors explaining this human particularity.[2] The authors measured the power of the sense of smell in 85 subjects after consumption of either alcoholic or non-alcoholic beverages. The differences between the groups were highly significant. The authors could conclude that "improved olfaction at low levels of alcohol supports the notion of an inhibitory mechanism obscuring true olfactory abilities".

When speaking with medical doctors and other health profes-sionals I find it easy and effective to refer to the "primitive reflexes". These reflexes are exhibited by normal newborn babies but disap-pear after a few weeks or months when the neocortex has reached a certain phase of development. Interestingly, older children and adults with pathological conditions such as cerebral palsy may retain these reflexes. Swimming reflexes belong to this framework. It is now well known that the capacity to adapt to immersion and make coordinated swimming movements when submerged is the rule among newborn babies. It disappears at around the age of three months. After that human beings are the only mammals who need to learn techniques to be able to swim with voluntary respiratory and muscular movements.

The Central Event

After disserting about the concept of neocortical inhibition, we don't need long developments to clarify the solution Nature found to make human birth possible and even occasionally easy. This solution is simply that the neocortex must reduce its activity. Even after thousands of years of socialisation of childbirth, including decades of masculinisation and medicalisation of the event, there are still some mothers and health professionals who have realised what is essential.

They know that when a woman can give birth easily by herself, without any pharmacological assistance, there is a time when she cuts herself off from our world, forgetting what she had been taught, forgetting her plans, and behaving in a way that usually would be considered unacceptable regarding a civilised woman, for example screaming or swearing. Some women can find themselves in the most unexpected, bizarre, often mammalian, primitive, quadrupedal postures. Interestingly there are anecdotes of women in hard labour complaining of odours nobody else could perceive: this is an eloquent symptom of reduced neocortical control.

This reduced neocortical activity is confirmed afterwards by a valuable study evaluating the well-known fact that many women forget details of what happened when they were in labour. Hundreds of women were interviewed about 10 days after giving birth. Those who had given birth by caesarean had a comparatively good recollection of many details.[3]

When this solution found by nature is understood, it becomes easy to analyse and summarise the basic needs of a labouring woman: a labouring woman needs to feel protected against all possible stimulations of her neocortex. The keyword is protection. Since language appears as a powerful neocortical stimulant, it is easy to reach the conclusion that silence is a basic need. The effects of light on the birth process have not been taken seriously until recently, when it appeared that melatonin, the "darkness hormone", is an essential birth hormone. This is why we'll multiply the opportunities to focus on this factor. While the effects of melatonin as an inhibitor of neocortical activity are already well understood, we'll see that this hormone has multiple targets during the birth process. From a practical perspective, we need to keep in mind that all attention-enhancing situations stimulate neocortical activity and therefore inhibit the birth process. Feeling observed is a typical example of this kind of situation: in other words, privacy appears as a basic need. The perception of a possible danger is another typical situation: in other words, to feel secure also appears as a basic need.

When the concept of neocortical inhibition appears as a key to explaining the particularities of human birth, extreme situations become less mysterious. We can learn, in particular, from women who can give birth easily. Before the age of modern pharmacology, it was well known that schizophrenic women usually gave birth quickly. Schizophrenic women behave in a way that is not culturally accept-able because their neocortical control is weak: today, brain imaging studies point to a reduction in grey matter volume in schizophrenia (particularly in the prefrontal cortex).[4] It has been also well known that "toxaemia" (the pregnancy disease now divided into pre-eclampsia and eclampsia) was usually associated with fast premature birth. Interestingly, according to "magnetic resonance spectroscopy", the brain of pre-eclamptic women does not receive the usual amount of blood, as if there was a narrowing of the carotid artery.[5] Anecdotes of women who gave birth while in a state of vegetative coma are also highly significant.

We must underline that we constantly use the terms "neocortical activity" and "neocortical inhibition" without referring to the extreme complexity of the human "new brain". It is on purpose. Precise technical terms such as "transient hypofrontality" or "deactivation of the frontal cortex" are not necessary to understand the essential.

Challenging Our Cultural Conditioning

By presenting childbirth in the light of modern physiology, we are challenging thousands of years of cultural conditioning. We present the birth process as an involuntary process under the control of primitive brain structures we share with the other mammals. As a general rule, one cannot help an involuntary process, but one can identify inhibitory factors. This is why, from a practical point of view, in terms of basic needs, the keyword is "protection". Since our point of departure has been the concept of neocortical inhibition, protection against language, light and attention-enhancing situations is given first place. If our point of departure had been the concept of adrenaline–oxytocin antagonism, we would have first mentioned protection from scary situations and low ambient temperature to explain that when mammals in general release emergency hormones of the adrenaline family, they cannot release oxytocin, the main birth hormone.

To present "protection" as a keyword is a preliminary, simple and concise way to challenge tradition. Since the beginning of the socialisation of childbirth, as an aspect of the domination of nature associated with the "Neolithic revolution", the basis of our cultural conditioning is that a woman has not the power to give birth by herself. She needs some kinds of cultural interferences. The dominant paradigm went through many phases, from the advent of midwifery and the most deep-rooted perinatal beliefs and rituals up to the current masculinisation and medicalisation of the birth environment. The current key words are eminently disempowering. They always focus on the active role of somebody else than mother and baby, the two obligatory actors in the birth drama. They are variants of the concepts of helping, guiding and controlling. The terms "coaching", used by groups promoting "natural childbirth", and "labour management", used in medical circles, imply the intervention of an expert, while the term "support" suggests that to give birth a woman needs energy brought by somebody else.

Today, one of the effects of a paradigm shift inspired by renewed physiological perspectives, and particularly the concept of neocortical inhibition, would be a better understanding of the pregnancy–parturition continuum. In other words, we can expect a future for the concept of "physiological birth preparation".

References

1. Betti L and Manica A (2018) Human variation in the shape of the birth canal is significant and geographically structured. *P R Soc B* Online at: doi.org/10.1098/rspb.2018.1807.
2. Endevelt-Shapira Y, Shushan S, Roth Y and Sobel N (2014) Disinhibition of olfaction: Human olfactory performance improves following low levels of alcohol. *Behav Brain Res* **272**:66–74. doi: 10.1016/j.bbr.2014.06.024.
3. Elkadry E, Kenton K, White P, *et al.* (2003) Do mothers remember key events during labor? *Am J Obstet Gynecol* **189**:195–200.
4. Meyer-Lindenberg A and Tost H (2014) Neuroimaging and plasticity in schizophrenia. *Restor Neurol Neurosc* **32(1)**:119–27. doi: 10.3233/RNN-139014.
5. Rutherford JM and Moody A (2003) Magnetic resonance spectroscopy in pre-eclampsia: Evidence of cerebral ischaemia. *BJOG* **110(4)**: 416–23.

Human Birth Preparation

Abstract

When the resistance to assimilating and popularising the concept of neocortical inhibition is overcome, it will be easier to go a step further and interpret some of the physiological maternal changes in late pregnancy. At the end of their pregnancies, many women claim that they are not as mentally sharp as usual (memory loss, poor concentration, renewed topics of interest, reduced and reoriented needs for socialisation). This deep-rooted empirical knowledge is now convincingly supported by brain imaging techniques, particularly those looking at gradual reductions in grey matter volumes in areas that play a key role in sociability. It is as if the need for privacy is already increasing before the labour starts. We must also give a great importance to the rising rates of melatonin (the "darkness hormone") during the pre-birth phase, since its release tends to reduce neocortical activity. Today, everybody has heard about oxytocin. In the near future, everybody will be aware of the relationship between oxytocin and the darkness hormone.

If we don't understand the birth process, we cannot understand how it is physiologically prepared.

In humans, characterised by a highly developed neocortex, there is an aspect of the physiological birth preparation that has remained ignored until now, although its symptoms and signs are well known. There are several obvious reasons for this cultural blindness. First, since the middle of the 20th century, the term "birth preparation" has often been used in the framework of methods designed by experts. Furthermore, as long as there is a strong resistance to assimilating and popularising the concept of neocortical inhibition, it is difficult to go a step further and fully understand some of the physiological maternal changes in late pregnancy.

From Empiric Knowledge to Brain Imaging Techniques

For a long time, it has been noticed that, at the end of their pregnancies, many women are not as mentally sharp as usual. They mention anecdotes of memory loss, and occasionally poor concentration. Their topics of interest become different. Their needs for socialisation may be reduced and reoriented.

This deep-rooted empirical knowledge is convincingly supported by imaging techniques. As early as 2003, an American study had observed that, in late pregnancy, there is a significant reduction of the blood flow in the large arteries going to the brain.[1] Significant decreases occur in both the middle and posterior cerebral arteries between 36 and 38 weeks of gestation. Unfortunately, there is no available data regarding brain blood flow during the very last days of pregnancy. According to a complementary study by the same authors, there is no reduction of the blood flow in the case of preeclampsia.[2] More recently, a Spanish and Dutch team has demonstrated that during pregnancy there are gradual reductions in grey matter volumes.[3] The observed volume reductions are not distributed randomly across the brain but are located in areas of the cortex that play a key role in sociability. It is as if the need for privacy is already increasing before the labour starts. Interestingly, 95.6% of the women could be correctly classified as pregnant using measures of grey matter volume changes. There were no changes in the grey matter volumes of the fathers, evidence for the selectivity of the changes for women undergoing pregnancy. Furthermore, brain changes were similarly affected regardless of means of conception (natural or medically assisted).

When raising questions about "the future of candles" we'll suggest that the rising rates of melatonin (the "darkness hormone") during the pre-birth phase might also be presented as a component of birth preparation since its release tends to reduce neocortical activity: the synergy between melatonin and GABA (inhibitory neurotransmitter) is an established fact.[4-6] The peak production of ALLO (allopregnanolone) by the placenta during the days preceding birth might also become an important chapter of physiological birth preparation. ALLO is a positive modulator of GABA.[7]

It is significant that, as long as birth physiology has not been understood as a chapter of brain physiology, studies of the hormone "relaxin" were among the only ones in the framework of what we call "physiological birth preparation" that attracted attention. As the word relaxin implies, one of the many demonstrated roles of this hormone is to prepare the mechanics of giving birth by relaxing pelvic ligaments and softening the pubic symphysis.

We must keep in mind that, in spite of technical and interpretational difficulties, altered memory and absentmindedness in pregnancy have been the topic of publications in a great diversity of scientific and medical journals. The common point between such studies is a widespread tendency to consider physiological changes during pregnancy only in the framework of preparation for motherhood. As long as there is a lack of interest in birth physiology, it is commonplace to forget that, between the time when a woman is pregnant and the phase of mother infant interaction, there is an acute and critical event, which is giving birth, and that this event needs to be physiologically prepared.

It is notable that the countless descriptions of what we present as symptoms and signs of birth preparation have attracted the attention of a diverse public. Some of them have directly reached health professionals involved in obstetrics,[8,9] others have reached psychiatrists,[10] others have reached mostly general practitioners,[11,12] other specialised physiologists.[13-15] Many have reached psychologists and psychotherapists, and had echoes in the media and the general public.

One can wonder why, in many such studies, it was difficult to confirm facts considered obvious and even established. The main reason is undoubtedly that researchers are not thinking in terms of birth preparation. This is why they are vague about the phases of pregnancy they are exploring. For example, in a huge study published in an authoritative journal of obstetrics,[9] a period as long as the last four months is presented as "late stage of pregnancy". Those who raise questions about physiological birth preparation would be more curious about the last four weeks and even the last four days! Another reason for discrepancies between the results is that memory has often been the main criterion explored by researchers. The point is that there are many kinds of memory: retrospective, prospective, short term, long term, spatial, verbal, visual, emotional, and also priming memory and working memory. When taking into account the point of view of mothers and the results of one particular study, it seems that an altered prospective memory (remembering to perform an act at the right time) is a frequent aspect of what is commonly called "baby brain".[16]

There are aspects of pre-labour behaviour that are not easily measured, and therefore evaluated through scientific methods. The high incidence of lost objects is still in the framework of empiric knowledge: there are countless anecdotes of women in late pregnancy who lost their keys, their mobile telephone, or their credit card. Some aspects of pre-labour behaviour justify the term "nesting instinct", since a nest is a protective structure built by certain animals to hold either eggs or the offspring or, occasionally, the animal itself. The content of a nest is cut off from the rest of the world. In humans, the urge to clean, tidy and organise the environment has been traditionally interpreted as a sign that labour and delivery are imminent. Our current understanding of birth physiology in humans suggests that in our species such behaviour cannot be dissociated from the framework of "birth preparation".

From an overview of what we learn from tradition, empiric knowledge and scientific knowledge, we can summarise a simple conclusion about the period of transition preceding labour: it is a phase of human life when down-to-earth preoccupations prevail over all the others.

To Whom It May Concern

From a practical perspective, the main question is: "Who must understand that before giving birth women need to live in peace and be protected against unnecessary intellectual stimulations?" The answer is that everybody is concerned, since everybody may occasionally have the opportunity to communicate with pregnant women. In other words, we are studying the evolution of cultural conditioning. However, in the context of the 21st century, we'll consider in particular several aspects of a radically renewed social environment.

The influence of the family has been dramatically modified within recent centuries and even decades. It is difficult to compare a traditional extended family, where pregnant women may feel protected among experienced mothers, with the small modern family structures. In the particular case of the nuclear family, the baby's father has often become a highly influential person. The extended family is more or less replaced by friends and colleagues, and by the informative role and intellectually stimulating effects of media and books. We must keep in mind that, until the middle of the 20th century, women were not reading books about pregnancy and birth.

In "The Age of Professions", some pregnant women are in a position to overcome the current cultural conditioning and take initiatives to try to satisfy what they feel as their basic needs. A significant example has been offered by Kylie Jenner, the famous American reality television star. After giving birth, she wrote: "I understand you're used to me bringing you along on all my journeys. My pregnancy was one I chose not to do in front of the world". There is food for thought in her attitude, because she is representative of a cultural milieu where the needs of pregnant women are usually ignored. We must recall that the USA has one of the lowest levels of maternity leave among the industrialised countries: women only have a right to a temporary and unpaid period of absence from employment immediately before and after giving birth. The contrast is enormous with a country such as Sweden, where parents can share 480 days of leave, including 420 paid by the Swedish Insurance company at a rate of 80% of the salary!

Since, with the advent of modern obstetrics, human pregnancies are highly medicalised, the focus should also be on the powerful influence of health professionals. On the day when it is understood how labour is physiologically prepared, the dominant style of prenatal care will be reconsidered: the results of sophisticated investigations and the risks associated with childbirth will not remain the central topics of conversation during a prenatal visit. Can we imagine a time when the main objective of health professionals is to interfere as little as possible in the shift towards down-to-earth preoccupations?

In the 1970s, I started to learn that the need for socialisation of pregnant women tends to be reoriented: I was able to observe the atmosphere of happiness that accumulated during singing encounters in the maternity unit at the Pithiviers hospital in France. These singing sessions probably had more positive effects on the birth process than additional series of medical tests.[17]

References

1. Zeeman GG, Hatab M and Twickler DM (2003) Maternal cerebral blood flow changes in pregnancy. *Am J Obstet Gynecol* **189(4)**: 968–72.

2. Zeeman GG, Hatab M and Twickler DM (2004) Increased cerebral blood flow in preeclampsia with magnetic resonance imaging. *Am J Obstet Gynecol* **191(4)**:1425–9.

3. Hoekzema E, Barba-Müller E, Pozzobon C, *et al.* (2016) Pregnancy leads to long-lasting changes in human brain structure. *Nat Neurosci* **20(2)**:287–96. doi: 10.1038/nn.4458.

4. Kivela A (1991) Serum melatonin during human pregnancy. *Acta Endocrinol (Copenh)* **124(3)**:233–7.

5. Tamura H, Nakamura Y, Terron MP, *et al.* (2008) Melatonin and pregnancy in the human. *Reprod Toxicol* **25(3)**:291–303. doi: 10.1016/j. reprotox.2008.03.005.

6. Nakamura Y, Tamura H, Kashida S, *et al.* (2001) Changes of serum melatonin level and its relationship to feto-placental unit during pregnancy. *J Pineal Res* **30(1)**:29–33.

7. Children's National Health System (2018) Placental ALLO levels rise during pregnancy and peak as fetuses approach full term. *ScienceDaily.* Online at: www.sciencedaily.com/releases/2018/05/180505091803.htm.

8. Sharp K, Brindle PM, Brown MW and Turner GM (1993) Memory loss during pregnancy. *Br J Obstet Gynaecol* **100(3)**:209–15.

9. Keenan PA, Yaldoo DT, Stress ME, *et al.* (1998) Explicit memory in pregnant women. *Am J Obstet Gynecol* **179(3 Pt 1)**:731–7.

10. Christensen H, Leach LS and Mackinnon A (2010) Cognition in pregnancy and motherhood: Prospective cohort study. *Br J Psychiatry* **196(2)**:126–32. doi: 10.1192/bjp.bp.109.068635.

11. Davies SJ, Lum JA, Skouteris H, *et al.* (2018) Cognitive impairment during pregnancy: A meta-analysis. *Med J Aust* **208(1)**:35–40.

12. de Groot RH, Vuurman EF, Hornstra G and Jolles J (2006) Differences in cognitive performance during pregnancy and early motherhood. *Psychol Med* **36(7)**:1023–32.

13. Shetty DN and Pathak SS (2002) Correlation between plasma neurotransmitters and memory loss in pregnancy. *J Reprod Med* **47(6)**:494–6.

14. Glynn LM (2010) Giving birth to a new brain: Hormone exposures of pregnancy influence human memory. *Psychoneuroendocrinology* **35(8)**:1148–55. doi: 10.1016/j.psyneuen.2010.01.015.
15. Henry JF and Sherwin BB (2012) Hormones and cognitive functioning during late pregnancy and postpartum: A longitudinal study. *Behav Neurosci* **126(1)**:73–85. doi: 10.1037/a0025540.
16. Rendell PG and Henry JD (2008) Prospective-memory functioning is affected during pregnancy and postpartum. *J Clin Exp Neuropsychol* **30(8)**:913–9. doi: 10.1080/13803390701874379.
17. Odent M (1984) *Birth Reborn*. Pantheon, New York.

The Future of Candles

Abstract

After presenting the concept of neocortical inhibition as a key to understanding the main particularities of human birth, we must raise questions about how the sensory functions connecting the brain and the environment work during the perinatal period, including the phase of preparation leading up to childbirth. There are several reasons to focus on the sense of sight. The first one is that melatonin, the "darkness hormone", appears today as synergetic with oxytocin in the brain and in the uterus as well. The second reason is that we are at a turning point in the history of artificial light. Until now incandescence had been the source of visible light. We are suddenly entering a new era, with the advent of LEDs (Light Emitting Diodes), based on the emission from semiconductors. From a practical perspective, the important point is that this new source of light has a powerful inhibitory effect on melatonin release, because it is rich in the blue part of the spectrum.

After presenting birth physiology in our species as a chapter of brain physiology, we must raise questions about how the sensory functions connecting the brain and the environment work during the phase of preparation for childbirth. Since melatonin — the "darkness hormone" — is now considered an essential birth hormone, working with oxytocin at several levels, we'll first focus on the sense of sight.

What Is Already Known

Let us recall that this hormone, released by the pineal gland, is involved in the regulation of day and night rhythms. In human adults, its synthesis and secretion increase shortly after the beginning of darkness, with maximum levels observed usually during the middle of the night (between 2 and 4 a.m.) and gradually decrease to basal daytime levels during the second half of the night. It is also well known that melatonin release is independently influenced by exposure to light. It has been confirmed that the inhibition of melatonin release is dependent on the intensity of light and the duration of exposure.[1-4] We even know about the kind of light that has the most powerful inhibitory effect on melatonin release: it is the blue part of the spectrum (between 446 and 477 nanometres).[5-7] This kind of knowledge is of paramount importance, since modern lifestyle is characterised by the widespread use of a new generation of artificial light.

We must keep in mind that from the time when our ancestors learned to control fire until recently, the only way to see in the dark was to use flames, which are the visible gaseous part of a fire. The use of candles, oil lamps, and petrol lanterns must be included in this framework. A new era started, at the beginning of the 19th century, when Sir Humphry Davy made the first incandescent electric lamp. This was followed by the age of incandescent light bulbs, that lasted until recently. The use of fluorescent lamps, which developed during the second part of the 20th century, is limited by health and safety issues. If a fluorescent lamp is broken, a small amount of mercury can contaminate the surrounding environment.

We are suddenly reaching a new phase in the use of artificial light with the advent of LEDs (Light Emitting Diodes). It is based on the light emission from semiconductors. The market of LEDs is projected to grow dramatically over the next decade. LEDs have many advantages over incandescent light sources, in particular lower energy consumption, and also long useful life, high degree of robustness and small size. With the advent of LEDs we suddenly need to raise new questions about the birth environment, since this modern source emits much more short wavelength light (the blue spectrum) than conventional sources. The basis of the current techniques is to first get blue light. Then white light is obtained by passing the blue rays through a yellow phosphor. The phosphor absorbs some of the blue and reradiates it as yellow: the combination of blue and yellow makes white. The point is that modern sources of light may have a powerful inhibitory effect on the release of melatonin, the darkness hormone. We are still in a phase of preliminary questions. This is why it is relevant to keep in mind the possible effects of factors often associated with exposure to modern artificial light. For example, being in front of a screen may be associated with an interactive, and therefore attention-enhancing situation, such as reading and answering a message.[8]

At such a turning point in the history of artificial light, Cornelia Gwinner, a French midwife, was curious enough to make a preliminary evaluation of the intensity and wavelengths of light commonly used in modern maternity units.[9] She had at her disposal a lux meter (measuring light intensity) and a spectrophotometer (measuring the brightness of the various portions of the light spectrum). She was able to conclude that today many women give birth in a light environment that is not appropriate. Therefore, we can ask the question: is there a future for candles in birthing places?

Meanwhile many properties of melatonin have been clarified. We have learned about the co-localisation of melatonin and oxytocin receptors in the central nervous system.[10] The synergy between melatonin and GABA (the main inhibitory neurotransmitter) is an established fact. Melatonin, as a component of the functional triad oxytocin–GABA–melatonin, undoubtedly has inhibitory effects on neocortical activity.[11-15] Although we are focusing on birth physiology as a chapter of brain physiology, we cannot ignore that the uterine muscle is directly sensitive to melatonin, since melatonin and oxytocin uterine receptors are synergetic.[16-20]

We must also keep in mind that the role of melatonin during the birth process is confirmed by its comparatively high concentration in the blood of babies "born with labour".[21] It is roughly twice the level among babies born by the vaginal route or by caesarean section during labour, compared with babies born by "pre-labour caesarean section". Let us open a parenthesis to underline the paramount importance of these findings: the protective anti-oxidative properties of melatonin are widely documented.

What We Need to Learn

To understand an important aspect of birth preparation, we need to learn from available data that have escaped notice as long as the concept of neocortical inhibition was not presented as a key to understanding human birth and as long as melatonin was not classified as a birth hormone. As early as 1991, Finnish researchers followed the fluctuations of blood melatonin concentrations among fifty-five healthy pregnant women.[22] They found a significant rise of melatonin in late pregnancy. The authors wondered if this rise was due to increased synthesis and secretion or retarded metabolism. More recently, a Japanese team confirmed the conclusions of the Finnish study.[23,24] They also found that the levels of melatonin decrease to non-pregnancy levels on the second day following birth. They completed their studies of blood concentrations in normal pregnancies by considering several particular cases, such as twin pregnancies and pre-eclampsia. In twin pregnancies the levels are higher than in singleton pregnancies, while they are comparatively low in the case of severe pre-eclampsia.

When combining the results of these Finnish and Japanese studies, we are in a position to claim that such demonstrations of an increased melatonin blood concentration in late pregnancy should be saved from oblivion. These little-known findings are still more valuable if introduced in the same framework as hard data provided by techniques of brain imaging. In further studies inspired by these preliminary results, it will be relevant to include precise data about the timing of the tests in relation to the spontaneous initiation of labour.

Smelling

When considering how the sensory functions connecting the brain and the environment work during the phase of birth preparation, there are reasons to focus on the sense of sight, since light has direct effects on neocortical activity. However, there are also reasons to consider the sense of smell, because there are well-known fluctuations in its power during pregnancy.

The sense of smell changes often start soon after conception. They are so well known that they may appear as the first signs of pregnancy. Some women suddenly react strongly to specific odours. This altered sense of smell may precede nausea and occasionally vomiting. Such symptoms during the first trimester of pregnancy are now considered adaptative.[25] It is almost a guarantee that the birth-weight will be at least equal to average. It is a sign of good placental activity.[26,27] It means that the placenta, as the advocate of the baby, "asks" the mother to eat just what she needs to survive. It is a way to reduce the risks of consuming too much harmful food at a critical phase of foetal development. Via a mechanism of compensation, the placenta is getting bigger. It is well known that vomiting pregnant women are at very low risk of miscarriage. Furthermore, it has been demonstrated that the risks of foetal abnormalities such as cleft lip[28] and anomalies of the penis (hypospadias)[29] are significantly reduced after pregnancies in which the mother has had episodes of vomiting.

Interestingly, traditional farmers knew about the advantages of food restriction in early pregnancy. Just after conception and for a limited period of time, they put ewes in poor pastures.

While the transitory increased sensitivity of olfaction in early pregnancy is well known, there has been until now a lack of interest in possible fluctuations of this sensory function in late pregnancy, in the phase of birth preparation. Once more, there is a need for studies that are precise in terms of timing and provide information about the number of days between a test and the spontaneous initiation of labour. The need for a new generation of studies seems obvious if we recall that the sense of smell is a typical example of physiological functions that are inhibited by neocortical activity.

References

1. Zeitzer JM, Dijk DJ, Kronauer R, et al. (2000) Sensitivity of human circadian pacemaker to nocturnal light: melatonin phase resetting and suppression. J Physiol **526(Pt 3)**:695–702.
2. McIntyre IM, Norman TR, Burrows GD and Armstrong SM (1989) Human melatonin suppression by light is intensity dependent. J Pineal Res **6(2)**:149–56.
3. Bojkowski CJ, Aldhous ME, English J, et al. (1987) Suppression of nocturnal plasma melatonin and 6-sulfatoxymelatonin by bright and dim light in man. Horm Metab Res **19(9)**:437–40.
4. Boyce P and Kennaway DJ (1987) Effects of light on melatonin production. Biol Psychiatry **22(4)**:473–8.
5. Brainard GC, Sliney D, Hanifin JP, et al. (2008) Sensitivity of the human circadian system to short wavelength (420 nm) light. J Biol Rhythms **23(5)**:379–86.
6. Kozaki T, Koga S, Toda N, et al. (2008) Effects of short wavelength control in polychromatic light sources on nocturnal melatonin secretion. Neurosci Lett **439(3)**:255–9.
7. Brainard GC, Hanifin JP, Greeson JM, et al. (2001) Action spectrum for melatonin regulation in humans: evidence for a novel circadian photoreceptor. J Neurosci **21(16)**:6405–12.

8. Smith LJ, King DL, Richardson C, *et al.* (2017) Mechanisms influencing older adolescents' bedtimes during videogaming: the roles of game difficulty and flow. *Sleep Med* **39**:70–6. doi: 10.1016/j. sleep.2017.09.002.

9. Cornélia Gwinner (2016) Influence de la lumière sur le processus de parturition humaine Revue de la littérature. *Gynécologie et obstétrique*. https://dumas.ccsd.cnrs.fr/dumas-01412390.

10. Wu YH, Zhou JN, Balesar R, *et al.* (2006) Distribution of MT1 melatonin receptor immunoreactivity in the human hypothalamus and pituitary gland: colocalization of MT1 with vasopressin, oxytocin and CRH. *J Comp Neurol* **499(6)**:897–910.

11. Wang F, Li J, Wu C, *et al.* (2003) The GABA(A) receptor mediates the hypnotic activity of melatonin in rats. *Pharmacol Biochem Behav* **74(3)**:573–8.

12. Meng T, Yuan S, Zheng Z, *et al.* (2015) Effects of endogenous melatonin on glutamate and GABA rhythms in the striatum of unilateral 6-hydroxydopamine-lesioned rats. *Neuroscience* **286**:308–15. doi: 10.1016/j.neuroscience.2014.11.062.

13. Marquez de Prado B, Castaneda TR, Galindo A, *et al.* (2000) Melatonin disrupts circadian rhythms of glutamate and GABA in the neostriatum of the aware rat: a microdialysis study. *J Pineal Res* **29(4)**:209–16.

14. Sato S, Yin C, Teramoto A, *et al.* (2008) Sexually dimorphic modulation of GABA(A) receptor currents by melatonin in rat gonadotropin-releasing hormone neurons. *J Physiol Sci* **58(5)**:317–22. doi: 10.2170/physiolsci.RP006208.

15. Sabihi S, Dong SM, Maurer SD, *et al.* (2017) Oxytocin in the medial prefrontal cortex attenuates anxiety: Anatomical and receptor specificity and mechanism of action. *Neuropharmacology* **125**:1–12. doi: 10.1016/j.neuropharm.2017.06.024.

16. Cohen M, Roselle D, Chabner B, *et al.* (1978) Evidence for a cytoplasmic melatonin receptor. *Nature* **274**:894–5.

17. Sharkey JT (2009) Melatonin Regulation of the Oxytocin System in the Pregnant Human Uterus. *Electronic Theses, Treatises and Dissertations.* Paper 1791. http://diginole.lib.fsu.edu/etd/1791.

18. Olcese J and Beesley S (2014) Clinical significance of melatonin receptors in the human myometrium. *Fertil Steril* **102(2)**:329–35. doi:10.1016/j.fertnstert.2014.06.020.

19. Schlabritz-Loutsevitch N, Hellner N, Middendorf R, *et al.* (2003) The human myometrium as a target for melatonin. *J Clin Endocrinol Metab* **88(2)**:908–13.

20. Sharkey JT, Puttaramu R, Word RA and Olcese J (2009) Melatonin synergizes with oxytocin to enhance contractility of human myometrial smooth muscle cells. *J Clin Endocrinol Metab* **94(2)**:421–7. doi: 10.1210/jc.2008-1723.

21. Bagci S, Berner AL, Reinsberg J, *et al.* (2012) Melatonin concentration in umbilical cord blood depends on mode of delivery. *Early Hum Dev* **88(6)**:369–73.

22. Kivela A (1991) Serum melatonin during human pregnancy. *Acta Endocrinol (Copenh)* **124(3)**:233–7.

23. Tamura H, Nakamura Y, Terron MP, *et al.* (2008) Melatonin and pregnancy in the human. *Reprod Toxicol* **25(3)**:291–303. doi: 10.1016/j.reprotox.2008.03.005.

24. Nakamura Y, Tamura H, Kashida S, *et al.* (2001) Changes of serum melatonin level and its relationship to feto-placental unit during pregnancy. *J Pineal Res* **30(1)**:29–33.

25. Flaxman SM and Sherman PW (2000) Morning sickness: a mechanism for protecting mother and embryo. *Q Rev Biol* **75(2)**:113–48.

26. Weigel RM and Weigel MM (1989) Nausea and vomiting of early pregnancy and pregnancy outcome. A meta-analytical review. *Br J Obstet Gynaecol* **96(11)**:1312–8.

27. Tierson FD, Olsen CL and Hook EB (1986) Nausea and vomiting of pregnancy and association with pregnancy outcome. *Am J Obstet Gynecol* **155(5)**:1017–22.

28. Czeizel AE, Sarhozi A and Wyszynski DF (2003) Protective effect of hyperemesis gravidarum for nonsyndromic oral clefts. *Obstet Gynecol* **101(4)**:737–44.

29. Akre O, Boyd HA and Ahlgren M (2008) Maternal and gestational risk factors for hypospadias. *Environ Health Perspect* **116(8)**:1071–6. doi: 10.1289/ehp.10791.

Chapter 5

Tackling an Epidemic

Abstract

Today, in many countries, about one quarter of human beings are born after labour induction. We can offer several interpretations for the high incidence of this medical procedure. The first one is that, until now, it has not been understood that labour induction is a way to shorten a probably crucial phase of human life. The second reason is that the dominant practices may be considered justified by the results of studies that exclusively use short term criteria. We must add that, in the case of prolonged pregnancy, it is commonplace to decide to induce labour without considering other factors than the time spent by the baby in the womb. It would be more rational to focus on placental functions. As long as placental functions are not declining, the need for action is disputable. From now on, it should be a major preoccupation among epidemiologists to explore the long-term consequences of being born after an interrupted phase of birth preparation.

In a 2018 French magazine interview, Karen Cleveland mentioned that the day before she gave birth to her first child, she had briefed her boss, the director of the CIA.

In 1975, in the series "Horizon", the television channel BBC 2 presented a documentary film — titled "A time to be born" — to investigate the growing incidence of labour induction. The practice has become increasingly widespread, at such a point it has now reached epidemic proportions.

After bringing together these two stories, we'll explore the possible links between them, taking into account that prolonged pregnancy is a frequent indication for labour induction: there are therefore reasons to focus on the issue of post-term birth. It appears, for people of my generation, that delayed spontaneous initiations of labour are more common today than in the middle of the 20th century. However, it is difficult to evaluate and to interpret this tendency because there have been fluctuations over the decades in the medical ways to interfere. Let us start from what is certain: today, for many reasons, the phase of birth preparation has been dramatically altered.

How to Protect a Crucial Phase of Human Life

After analysing some well-documented components of this phase of human life, in particular the shift towards down-to-earth preoccupations and a reduced and reoriented need for socialisation, we must go a step further. Now we have to consider how the phase of birth preparation can be protected. The way we phrase appropriate questions is more important than the preliminary recipes we might suggest.

An example of a broad and useful question that must be adapted to particular cases is: how to protect a woman in late pregnancy against useless intellectual stimulations. In the 1970s, in the Pithiviers hospital (France), we had this question in mind when inviting pregnant women to come and sing around the piano. At that time, we were not referring to sophisticated theoretical considerations. There was an atmosphere of happiness when these women were singing and occasionally dancing together. They could satisfy their reoriented social needs by sharing their down-to-earth preoccupation with other pregnant women and young mothers and their newborn babies. I was tacitly thinking that such sessions probably had more positive effects on the way women give birth than "serious" conversations about, for example, the risks of prolonged pregnancies, the size of the baby's head according to the last ultrasound scan, or the need for iron tablets.

Another example of a useful question is: how to protect women in late pregnancy against light pollution? This is a topic we cannot evade, at a time when melatonin, the darkness hormone, appears as an important birth hormone, since its release is inhibited by light, particularly several kinds of artificial light, and since an increased melatonin blood concentration may be considered a component of birth preparation. Light pollution is becoming a serious issue for many reasons: disruptions of ecosystems, effects on astronomy, aesthetic considerations and also health effects. We have recently learned, through photos of Earth from outer space, that true darkness has disappeared: a turning point in the history of the planet.[1]

Many possible adverse health effects of artificial light must be considered. The most valuable epidemiological studies looked at the risk of cancer, particularly breast cancer, among women who work at night.[2-5] These women experience sleep deprivation, disruptions of the day and night cycle, and exposure to light at night. The most plausible culprit is the lack of melatonin as a cancer protective agent. Other studies of over-illumination or improper spectral composition looked at headache incidence, worker fatigue, sexual dysfunctions, mood and anxiety.

Interestingly, although the epidemic of labour induction is topical, the plausible effects of light pollution in late pregnancy have not yet inspired scientific research. However, from a practical perspective, we already have good reasons to wonder how, in the period preceding birth, women might protect themselves. There is no risk of suggesting that expectant mothers might try to moderate exposure to artificial light and, in particular, to reduce the time spent in front of computer and television screens. If necessary, they might also occasionally wear amber glasses to block the blue part of the spectrum. In terms of public health, one can imagine a time when it will be considered necessary to establish the safe limits of the so-called "blue light hazard", taking into account the particular case of the perinatal period. Once more, at the present time, the point is not to offer recipes, it is to phrase appropriate new questions.

The Risk of Overestimation

In an attempt to interpret the current epidemic of labour induction, we have focused on two probable factors that are related. One is the excess of intellectual stimulation, the other one is light pollution. These are factors that have not been previously considered. We are aware of the risk of overestimating their comparative importance, while forgetting previously acquired knowledge. We must keep in mind that other aspects of modern lifestyles undoubtedly alter the pre-birth period.

It is well known that, among mammals in general, stress hormones inhibit physiological functions related to reproduction. In a wild environment, if a female ready to give birth has perceived the presence of a predator, she releases hormones of the adrenaline family that give her the energy to fight or to escape: the birth process is postponed. A well-known experiment has demonstrated that a cow has no milk ejection reflex if a cat has been put on her back. Among humans, we can guess that couples cannot make love during an earthquake or a bombardment. It is as if the need to survive as an individual is a priority. In emergency situations, the need to survive by reproduction is postponed.

Such considerations lead us to wonder if modern pregnant women release more stress hormones than women from previous generations, although the vital risks associated with childbirth have dramatically decreased within some decades. Their physiological states are undoubtedly influenced by the amount and the nature of information they are exposed to, the anticipation of being in unfamiliar environments among unfamiliar persons when giving birth, and probably by many aspects of a renewed conditioning. If, today, women have more opportunities to release stress hormones than in the past, we should expect alterations of the initiation of labour.

Since the perinatal period is highly medicalised, we cannot ignore the effects of medical strategies on the current epidemic. It is commonplace today to decide to induce labour without taking into account other factors than the gestational age of the foetus. It would be more rational to focus on placental functions. As long as placental functions are not declining, the need for action is disputable.

When I was practicing in a hospital an hour from Paris, we were taking advantage of what a research laboratory at "La Faculté de Médecine de Paris" (laboratory of Professor Max Jayle) could offer. They could easily and quickly evaluate the urine concentrations of hormones such as human placental lactogen, placental growth hormone and human chorionic gonadotrophin. We just had to bring a sample of urine from a woman who had a prolonged pregnancy and, soon after by telephone, we were given the results, which usually were "good placental function". This non-invasive test could be repeated. I used to associate this laboratory test with amnioscopies, a practice that is now forgotten.[6] An amnioscope is a thin endoscope that is easily introduced into the cervix. As long as the amniotic fluid appears clear with some flocks of vernix, it is almost a guarantee that the placental functions are good enough. It is significant of the current dominant way of thinking that today it is not commonplace to repeat ultrasound scans to evaluate the amount of amniotic fluid in the case of prolonged pregnancies. It is an indirect way to get some clues about placental functions.

Thanks to this strategy I learned that foetal distress related to post maturity is possible, but not common. The main lesson is that some foetuses need a longer time than others to be mature. Babies are occasionally born covered with vernix caseosa, and therefore don't look post mature, after spending much more than nine months in the womb, while others have a dry skin when born before the official due date. It is as if we need to rediscover ancient empiric knowledge. The authoritative academic book by Jacques Gelis about childbirth in rural Europe between the 16th and the 19th century was titled "L'arbre et le fruit" (the tree and the fruit).[7] This title was a reference to the widespread belief that a baby in the womb is like a fruit on a tree. If we pick up a fruit that is not ripe it will not taste good and it will get spoiled very quickly.[8]

An increased interest in the placenta as an endocrine gland should be an important step in the control of the epidemic of labour induction.

By using the term "epidemic" we associate the skyrocketing rates of labour induction with a negative connotation. This issue must not be marginalised, since in many countries about one quarter of human beings are born after labour induction, and even one third in some hospitals. It is plausible that the prevalence of labour induction will not decrease in the near future, since authoritative medical journals publish studies comparing induction at 39 weeks and "expectative management".[9] Of course, such studies only consider short-term criteria. As a first step, epidemiologists might introduce middle-term effects on maternal health. For example, postpartum depression is topical, because apparently more frequent than ever. There are theoretical reasons to wonder if the elimination or the shortening of the phase of birth preparation by labour induction is a risk factor. A huge study involved all women who gave birth in Sweden from 1997 to 2008.[10] Labour induction was not taken into account. However, since the diagnosis of gestational diabetes is usually associated with comparatively high rates of labour induction, it is notable that this diagnosis appeared as a highly significant risk factor.

It should become a major preoccupation among epidemiologists to try to explore the long-term consequences of being born after induced labour. Until now, an exploration of the Primal Health Research database (www.primalhealthresearch.com) through the keyword "labour induction" leads to only two dozen studies. Most of them are related to the risks of autism. It seems that the main motivation of researchers has been to explore possible risk factors for autism rather than long-term non-specific consequences of labour induction.

The generation of epidemiological studies we are expecting will have to overcome obvious difficulties. One of them will be to dissociate the effects of a shortened phase of birth preparation and the specific effects of drugs used for labour induction.

References

1. *NASA* (2012) NASA-NOAA Satellite Reveals New Views of Earth at Night. Press release 12–422. https://www.nasa.gov/mission_pages/NPP/news/earth-at-night.html.
2. Schernhammer ES and Schulmeister K (2004) Melatonin and cancer risk: does light at night compromise physiologic cancer protection by lowering serum melatonin levels? *Br J Cancer* **90(5)**:941–3.
3. Davis S and Mirick DK (2006) Circadian disruption, shift work and the risk of cancer: a summary of the evidence and studies in Seattle. *Cancer Causes Control* **17(4)**:539–45.
4. Reiter RJ, Tan DX, Korkmaz A, et al. (2007) Light at night, chronodisruption, melatonin suppression, and cancer risk: a review. *Crit Rev Oncog* **13(4)**:303–28.
5. Dumont M, Lanctôt V, Cadieux-Viau R and Paquet J (2012) Melatonin production and light exposure of rotating night workers. *Chronobiol Int* **29(2)**:203–10. doi: 10.3109/07420528.2011.647177.
6. Odent M (2006) Should midwives re-invent the amnioscope? *Midwifery Today* **80:7**, 66.
7. Jacques Gélis (1984) *L'arbre et le fruit*. Fayard. Paris.
8. Odent M (2004) The tree and the fruit: routine versus selective strategies in postmaturity. *Midwifery Today* **72**:18–9. https://midwiferytoday.com/mt-articles/the-tree-and-the-fruit/.

9. Grobman WA, Rice MM, Reddy UM, *et al.* (2018) Labor induction versus expectant management in low-risk nulliparous women. *N Engl J Med* **379(6)**:513–23. doi: 10.1056/NEJMoa1800566.
10. Silverman ME, Reichenberg A, Savitz DA, *et al.* (2017) The risk factors for postpartum depression: A population-based study. *Depress Anxiety* **34(2)**:178–87. doi: 10.1002/da.22597.

Pre-Labour Caesareans

Abstract

Birth by caesarean before labour starts may be presented as a quasi-experimental association of an interrupted phase of birth preparation, foetal stress deprivation and microbial deprivation. On the day when the phase of physiological birth preparation is topical, and when the particularities of babies born in states of stress deprivation and microbial deprivation are studied in depth, there will probably be an accumulation of new reasons to avoid whenever it is possible the practice of pre-labour caesareans. If we add that, for obvious reasons, caesareans performed in a context of real emergency are associated with comparatively poor outcomes, there is a future for the concept of "in-labour non-emergency caesareans".

A pre-labour caesarean section is another frequent way to interrupt the phase of birth preparation. While we had reasons to associate the issues of labour induction and pharmacological assistance, we have in the same way, reasons to associate birth by pre-labour caesarean and stress deprivation.

In the framework of our cultural conditioning, "stress" has a negative connotation: we must avoid stressful situations. Meanwhile, in the current scientific context, it appears that stress hormones have multiple roles to play and the concept of "stress deprivation" has recently emerged in scholarly articles. Birth by pre-labour caesarean may be presented as an extreme and quasi-experimental example of stress deprivation.[1]

It has been understood for a long time that pre-labour caesarean is a risk factor for respiratory difficulties in the neonatal period, and that the risks are dependent on the gestational age: differences in the quality of the respiratory functions are detectable when comparing pre-labour births at 38 and 39 weeks.[2] One of the interpretations is that the foetus participates in the initiation of labour, probably through the release of surfactant, when its lungs have reached a certain degree of maturity.[3] Furthermore, the roles of maternal and foetal stress hormones are well known. The effects of maternal corticosteroids on foetal lung maturation have had practical implications for several decades. Labour implies the action of beta-endorphin (releasers of prolactin, which participate in lung maturation).[4] Labour also implies the release of the foetal noradrenaline, probably one of the main factors participating in lung maturation.

Recent Human Studies

The important point is that the multiple effects of stress deprivation among babies born by pre-labour C-section have been underestimated until recently. For example, it has been demonstrated that, under the effect of noradrenaline, the sense of smell has reached a high degree of maturity at birth among babies born by in-labour C-section or via the vaginal route. The principle of a Swedish experiment was to expose babies to an odour for 30 minutes shortly after birth and then to test them for their response to this odour at the age of three or four days.[5] Since the concentrations of foetal stress hormones (noradrenaline) had been evaluated, it was possible to conclude that foetal noradrenaline released during labour is involved in the maturation of the sense of smell. We must emphasise the paramount role of the sense of smell immediately after birth.

I had already mentioned in the 1970s that the sense of smell is the main guide towards the nipple as early as the first hour following birth.[6,7] It has been demonstrated that it is mostly through the sense of smell that the newborn baby can identify its mother (and, to a certain extent, that the mother can identify her baby).

There has been recently an accumulation of data regarding the effects of caesarean births according to their timing.

Among such studies, we must mention the evaluation of adiponectin concentration in cord blood of healthy babies born at term. The concentration of this agent involved in fat metabolism is significantly lower after pre-labour caesarean compared with in-labour caesarean or vaginal route.[8] These data suggest a mechanism according to which stress deprivation at birth might be a risk factor for obesity in childhood and adulthood.

In the framework of human studies, we must recall the evaluations of the concentrations of melatonin in the cord blood. It is low after pre-labour births.[9] This is an important point, since melatonin has protective anti-oxidative properties. Furthermore, it confirms that the "darkness hormone" is involved in the birth process. This is one of the reasons why the role of melatonin during labour is topical, at a time when we are learning about a synergy between its uterine receptors and oxytocin receptors.

In general, a baby born after a pre-labour caesarean is physiologically different from the others. For example, babies born pre-labour tend to have a lower body temperature than the others during the first 90 minutes following birth.[10]

Animal Experiments

In spite of possible inter-species differences, we must seriously consider animal experiments suggesting that the stress of labour influences brain development. Such is the case of studies demonstrating that the birth process in mice triggers the expression of a protein (uncoupled protein 2) that is important for the hippocampus development.[11] Let us recall that, among humans, the hippocampus is a major component of the limbic system. It has been compared to an "orchestra conductor" directing brain activity. It has also been presented as a kind of physiological GPS system, helping us navigate while also storing memories in space and time: the work of three scientists who studied this important function of the hippocampus has been recognised by the award of the 2014 Nobel Prize in physiology and medicine. This is also the case of studies with rats suggesting that oxytocin-induced uterine contractions reverse the effects of the important neurotransmitter GABA: this primary excitatory neurotransmitter becomes inhibitory.[12] If uterine contractions affect the neurotransmitter systems of rats during an important phase of brain development, why wouldn't the same thing occur in humans?

The Future

Other effects of pre-labour caesareans will probably appear in the near future. It seems that the prevalence of placenta praevia is significantly increased only in the case of a pregnancy following a pre-labour cesarean.[13] There is already an accumulation of data confirming the negative effect of pre-labour caesarean on breastfeeding, particularly at the phase of initiation of lactation.[14,15] We cannot ignore data regarding the milk microbiome. There are significant differences between the milk of mothers who gave birth by pre-labour caesarean and those who gave birth by in-labour caesarean or the vaginal route.[16] These results suggest that an artificially shortened phase of birth preparation might alter the process of microbial transmission to milk. Similar differences were found by a Canadian study of the gut flora of four-month-old babies.[17] Joanna Holbrook and her team, in Singapore, suggest interpretations for these surprising data. They collected faecal samples from 75 babies at the age of 3 days, 3 weeks, 3 months and 6 months. It appears that, apart from the route of birth and exposure to antibiotics, a shortened duration of pregnancy tends to delay the maturation of the gut flora: one week more or less in the duration of pregnancy is associated with significant differences: a pre-labour caesarean implies the association of all the known factors that can delay the maturation of the gut flora.[18]

In the future, when the phase of physiological birth preparation is topical, and when the particularities of newborn babies born in a state of stress deprivation are studied in depth, there will probably be an accumulation of new reasons to avoid whenever it is possible the practice of pre-labour caesareans. In many situations, a planned caesarean may be delayed until the onset of labour. This is the case, for example, of women who have expressed a severe fear of childbirth. The prevalence of "tocophobia" has dramatically increased during the past two decades.[19] It is an inevitable topic since, according to recent estimations, the prevalence of this kind of phobia might be in the region of 14%.

If we add that, for obvious reasons, caesareans performed in a context of real emergency are associated with comparatively poor outcomes, there is a future for the concept of "in-labour non-emergency caesareans".

References

1. Odent M (2015) Stress deprivation in the perinatal period. *Midwifery Today* **116**:25–7.
2. Glavind J and Uldbjerg N (2015) Elective cesarean delivery at 38 and 39 weeks: neonatal and maternal risks. *Curr Opin Obstet Gynecol* **27(2)**:121–7. doi: 10.1097/GCO.0000000000000158.
3. Condon JC, Jeyasuria P, Faust JM and Mendelson CR (2004) Surfactant protein secreted by the maturing mouse fetal lung acts as a hormone that signals the initiation of parturition. *Proc Natl Acad Sci USA* **101(14)**:4978–83.

4. Hauth JC, Parker CR Jr, MacDonald PC, *et al.* (1978) A role of fetal prolactin in lung maturation. *Obstet Gynecol* **51(1)**:81–8.
5. Varendi H, Porter RH and Winberg J (2002) The effect of labor on olfactory exposure learning within the first postnatal hour. *Behav Neurosci* **116(2)**:206–11.
6. Odent M (1977) The early expression of the rooting reflex. *Proc 5th Int Con Psychosom Obstet Gynaecol* 1117–19. Academic Press, London.
7. Odent M (1978) L'expression précoce du réflexe de fouissement. In: *Les cahiers du nouveau-né* **12**:169185.
8. Hermansson H, Hoppu U and Isolauri E (2014) Elective caesarean section is associated with low adiponectin levels in cord blood. *Neonatology* **105**:172–4. doi: 10.1159/000357178.
9. Bagci S, Berner AL, Reinsberg J, *et al.* (2012) Melatonin concentration in umbilical cord blood depends on mode of delivery. *Early Hum Dev* **88(6)**:369–73.
10. Christensson K, Siles C, Cabrera T, *et al.* (1993) Lower body temperature in infants delivered by caesarean section than in vaginally delivered infants. *Acta Paediatr* **82(2)**:128–31.
11. Simon-Areces J, Dietrich MO, Hermes G, *et al.* (2012) Ucp2 induced by natural birth regulates neuronal differentiation of the hippocampus and related adult behavior. *PLoS ONE* **7(8)**:e42911. doi: 10.1371/journal.pone.0042911.
12. Tyzio R, Cossart R, Khalilov I, *et al.* (2006) Maternal oxytocin triggers a transient inhibitory switch in GABA signaling in the fetal brain during delivery. *Science* **314**:1788–92.
13. Downes KL, Hinkle SN, Sjaarda LA, *et al.* (2015) Prior prelabor or intrapartum cesarean delivery and risk of placenta previa. *Am J Obstet Gynecol* **212(5)**:669e1–669e6.
14. Prior E, Santhakumaran S, Gale S, *et al.* (2012) Breastfeeding after cesarean delivery: A systematic review and meta-analysis of world literature. *Am J Clin Nutr* **95(5)**:1113–35. doi: 10.3945/ajcn.111.030254.
15. Zanardo V, Savolna V, Cavallin F, *et al.* (2012) Impaired lactation performance following elective cesarean delivery at term: role of maternal levels of cortisol and prolactin. *J Matern Fetal Neonatal Med* **25(9)**:1595–8. doi: 10.3109/14767058.2011.648238.

16. Cabrera-Rubio R, Collado MC, Laitinen K, *et al*. (2012) The human milk microbiome changes over lactation and is shaped by maternal weight and mode of delivery. *Am J Clin Nutr* **96(3)**:544–51. doi: 10.3945/ajcn.112.037382.

17. Azad MB, Konya T, Maugham H, *et al*. (2013) Gut microbiota of healthy Canadian infants: profiles by mode of delivery and infant diet at 4 months. *CMAJ* **185(5)**:385–94. doi.org/10.1503/cmaj.121189.

18. Dogra S, Sakwinska O, Soh S, *et al*. (2015) Dynamics of infant gut microbiota are influenced by delivery mode and gestational duration and are associated with subsequent adiposity. *mBio* **6(1)**:e02419-14. doi: 10.1128/mBio.02419-14.

19. O'Connell MA, Leahy-Warren P, Khashan AS, *et al*. (2017) Worldwide prevalence of tocophobia in pregnant women: systematic review and meta-analysis. *Acta Obstet Gynecol Scand* **96(8)**:907–20. doi: 10.1111/aogs.13138.

Chapter 7

Eclampsia: Lessons from a Human Disease

Abstract

Since this pregnancy disease is usually considered specific to Homo, it is an obligatory topic for all students of human nature. One of the objectives of this chapter is to illustrate the concept of an interdisciplinary perspective.

The phase of birth preparation may be altered by pathological conditions, particularly eclampsia. Since authentic eclampsia (with convulsions) has become rare in developed countries (even before the age of medicalised prevention), the focus is usually on "preeclampsia" and the topics of interest are dominated by placental implantation. To shed light on several puzzling aspects of eclampsia, we should first consider fluctuations in the prevalence of the disease and emphasise that the orders of magnitude are not the same in poor populations with cereal based diets compared to a high standard of living. Furthermore, we suggest that eclampsia should be studied in the framework of maternal-foetal conflicts. The nature and the expression of these conflicts among different species of mammals depend on the nutritional priorities during the early phase of development. Among humans, it appears that the priority is to satisfy the nutritional needs of the developing brain.

Considerations about nutritional needs suggest questions about the prevalence of specifically human diseases before and after the advent of agriculture.

Since this disease is usually considered specific to Homo, it is an obligatory topic for all students in human nature.

After analysing many components of modern lifestyle, including medical practices, that alter or interrupt the phase of physiological birth preparation, we must also consider eclampsia. Eclampsia, which had already been described by Hippocrates, is characterised by seizures during the second half of pregnancy. It can occasionally occur during the hours or days following birth. It is life threatening for mother and baby. It is notable that the prevalence of eclampsia has been continuously decreasing in developed countries throughout the 20th century. Medical advances are not sufficient to explain how eclampsia became rare in many parts of the world, since there was no effective preventive treatment, apart from interruption of pregnancy, until the very recent widespread use of magnesium sulphate and aspirin. Interpretations must therefore be found in the framework of radical changes in lifestyle. What kind of changes should we consider?

Different Orders of Magnitude

Today, when referring to the prevalence of eclampsia, we must first realise that the order of magnitude is not the same in developing countries compared with high standard of living populations. In wealthy countries the prevalence may be as low as 0.03%: precise data have been provided by British and Japanese statistics, in particular.[1,2] In low income populations, on the other hand, the prevalence may be in the region of 5%, whatever the continent, even when magnesium sulphate, aspirin and caesarean sections are available. This is the case, for example, of Bangladesh in Asia, Burkina Faso in Africa, and Haiti in America. According to a study conducted at Dhaka Medical College and Hospital, Bangladesh, among the 32,999 women who were admitted between 1998 and 2000, 9% had eclampsia convulsions. Among them, the rate of maternal deaths was

8.6%.[3] At the University hospital of Ouagadougou (Burkina Faso), 203 cases of eclampsia for 6,063 births were identified between 1st April 2013 and 31st March 2014, that to say a prevalence of 3.3%. The maternal mortality rate was 6.4%. The perinatal mortality rate was 31.5% of the cases.[4] In Haiti, the prevalence of eclampsia is also among the highest in the world, and has probably increased after the historical 2010 earthquake, but there is a lack of valuable statistical data, in spite of the presence of "Doctors without Borders" and the United Nations stabilisation mission.

Modern medical practices, which have a limited preventive effect where eclampsia is concerned, cannot explain why in some parts of the world "the disease of theories" is one hundred times more common than in others. This fact should be a point of departure to unveil the roots of this specifically human condition. We must first wonder what countries such as Bangladesh, Burkina Faso and Haiti have in common. The answer is apparently simple. In the countries where eclampsia is common, the rates of malnutrition among women are the highest in the world and there is a lack of diversity in their cereal-based diets.

When keeping in mind these comparisons between countries with different lifestyles, and also after recalling that this pregnancy disease became less and less common throughout the 20th century in wealthy countries, we may wonder why the medical and scientific literature is not submerged by studies focusing on nutritional factors. The reasons are obvious: researchers are trained in wealthy countries where eclampsia has almost completely disappeared. They share the dominant preoccupations of our time in the influential medical community. They also share the dominant theoretical framework. They focus on the warning state called pre-eclampsia, losing interest in the real eclampsia, and they usually start from the narrow viewpoint that studying this condition is roughly the equivalent of studying faulty placental implantation. They have difficulties going beyond the well-accepted model according to which in a first stage abnormal implantation results in reduced placental perfusion and in a second stage there is an altered release of placental factors into the maternal circulation.

Learning from Isolated Pioneers

However, it is worth recalling that after the time when the theory of toxins was dismissed and the word "toxaemia" gradually replaced, and before the wide use of the concept of pre-eclampsia and the exclusive focus on faulty placental implantation, several more or less isolated pioneers had understood the paramount importance of nutritional factors. This is the case of Adolphe Pinard (the inventor of the obstetrical stethoscope). He had huge experience, in his "Lying-in hospital" in Paris, of pregnancies among poor malnourished single mothers, who were at high risks of eclampsia. In an historical conference in 1900, he just explained that giving them a lot of milk every day had been a simple way to control the epidemic.[5]

More recently, in the USA, immediately after World War II, Robert Ross published a report in an authoritative medical journal showing that there was a high eclampsia incidence among the malnourished poor populations of the Southern American states.[6] Soon after, in another authoritative medical journal, James Ferguson published a similar report focusing on the severe malnutrition of eclamptic women in rural Mississippi.[7] At the same phase of medical history, the most spectacular and convincing report was published in The Lancet.[8] An intensive nutrition education programme had been introduced in the Sydney Women's hospital. This programme was based on frequent lectures given by the medical superintendent and the dietitian to women all through their pregnancies. The objective was to promote a "high-protein, high-vitamin, and low-carbohydrate diet" (in practice to reduce the amount of cereals) and to correct the most usual nutritional deficiencies in Melbourne at that time. On March 25, 1951, this maternity unit (about 5,000 booked pregnant women a year) had completed for the first time a year without a single case of eclampsia. Robert Hamlin, the author of the report, enthusiastically wrote that "these lectures had reaped results far in excess of what was expected of them when they were begun in 1948". He dared to use the term "eradication of eclampsia" long before the age of magnesium sulphate, aspirin, synthetic oxytocin and even safe techniques of caesarean sections. We must keep in mind that it was not until the 1990s that major controlled studies demonstrated the superiority of magnesium sulphate over other anticonvulsants. Robert Hamlin had introduced his report by recalling the authoritative point of view of O'Donel Browne in 1950, when he was the "Master of the Rotunda Hospital" in Dublin: "Antenatal supervision seems to be a poor safeguard against fulminating tox-aemia". If we read between the lines we understand that it is more important to multiply the opportunities to talk about nutrition than to multiply the medicalised visits.

After this series of valuable reports in the authoritative medical literature in the middle of the 20th century, we can only mention the popular books by Tom Brewer, in the USA. In his books and his conferences, Tom Brewer has encouraged pregnant women to consume without any restriction food such as eggs, cheese, dairy products in general, and meat. The focus was on the need for pro-tein and calories. Interestingly, Tom Brewer repeatedly emphasised that during the last eight weeks of foetal life "brain development is occurring at the most rapid rate ever". However, in the context of 1977, he was not in a position to give importance to the specific nutritional needs of the developing brain, particularly in terms of fatty acids and iodine.[9]

In the age of pre-eclampsia, the interest for nutrition has van-ished. There have been countless studies of risk factors such as prior hypertension, older age, diabetes mellitus and obesity, and pregnancies with different procreators, but the nutritional factors are not investigated any more, apart from the possible effects of isolated nutrients, particularly calcium and vitamin E, C or D. New ways to classify pre-eclamptic states have been suggested in relation to the time when the first signs of the condition where detected. Even the concept of pre-eclampsia might be gradually replaced by the term "Hypertensive disorders in pregnancy", while variants of the syndrome are described, such as the "HELLP syndrome", which combines red blood cell breakdown, impaired liver function and low blood platelet count. New predictive tests are continuously offered and evaluated. The objective of an impressive number of published studies is to identify in early pregnancy women who should take aspirin.

One can wonder if some aspects of the modern lifestyle, particularly the sudden expansion of veganism, could inspire a new generation of epidemiological research taking nutritional factors into account. The point is not to express premature opinions about such a sudden and widespread phenomenon.

We can just anticipate that epidemiologists will have to overcome technical difficulties. The main difficulty will be to eliminate the effects of associated factors and to provide valuable conclusions from studies of self-selected groups: veganism is associated with other aspects of lifestyle. Furthermore, it will be difficult to take into account that there are many kinds of vegans. However, we can at least claim that, theoretically, a well-planned vegan diet in pregnancy can satisfy the nutritional needs of the fast-developing foetal brain, a priority in our species. Such a diet can easily provide an appropriate amount of the parent molecule of the omega-3 family of fatty acids and of the catalysts of the metabolic pathway of this family. Let us recall that the brain is a mostly fatty organ, and that the developing brain has specific needs, particularly in terms of very long chain omega-3 fatty acids. We must also take into account that, as a general rule, vegans don't consume significant amounts of pure sugar, alcohol, trans fatty acids of refined oils and margarine, and other blocking agents of the metabolic pathways of unsaturated fatty acids. As for iodine, which is also essential for brain development and brain functions, it can be provided by a vegan diet, particularly by seaweeds. There is an urgent and vital need for valuable studies of the vitamin B12 status (and the development) of vegan infants.

Meanwhile, while anticipating a renewed interest for nutrition in pregnancy, most studies of the human disease eclampsia are related to placental perfusion, vascular resistance and oxidative stress. From a therapeutic perspective, one of the dominant objectives of current research is to silence circulating endothelial growth factor receptors of placental origin. In spite of an intense publishing activity, many aspects of the disease remain mysterious.

Interspecies Comparisons of Maternal–Foetal Conflicts

It is in such a context that I have studied the human disease eclampsia from an interspecies perspective in the framework of the concept of mother–offspring conflicts.

It is well understood that, among mammals in general, mother and foetus do not carry identical sets of genes: in the child there are maternally derived genes and also paternal sets of genes. In other words, the harmony of interests between mother and foetus cannot be complete. There are obvious reasons for conflicts. Until now the dominant preoccupations have been unidirectional: why the mother's immune system doesn't destroy the developing foetus? Any analysis of a conflict between two individuals should imply a bidirectional perspective. This is why we must keep in mind that one of the roles of the placenta is to be the "advocate of the baby": as an endocrine gland, the placenta can manipulate maternal physiology for foetal benefit. A maternal disease occurs when the demands of the foetus(es) via the placenta exceed what the mother can provide without creating her own imbalances.

The nature, the timing and the expression of maternal–foetal conflicts among different species of mammals depend on the nutritional priorities during the perinatal phase of development.

For example, where ewes and does are concerned, veterinarians use the terms "pregnancy disease" or "pregnancy toxaemia". Among these herbivorous mammals the foetus is supplied almost entirely by glucose, consuming 40% of the blood sugar produced by the mother. The disease occurs in late pregnancy. It is more common in the case of thin ewes pregnant with multiple foetuses. It is characterised by a destabilisation of the glycaemia that leads to fat catabolism (this disease has also been called "lambing ketosis"). Treatment is based on the administration of glucose. Among dogs and cats, the so-called eclampsia or perinatal tetany is related to hypocalcaemia (its expression usually starts after the birth). Of course, where these carnivorous species are concerned, the priority at the end of pregnancy and at the beginning of lactation is the development of the bones of the offspring, which are much more mature at birth than the bones of other mammals. Treatment is based on the intravenous administration of calcium.

Interspecies comparisons encourage us to raise new questions concerning the potential for gestational conflicts among humans, characterised by a gigantic brain. The spectacular brain growth spurt during the second half of foetal life is a specifically human trait. A conflict between the demands of the foetus and what the mother can provide without creating her own imbalances leads us to consider first the needs of the developing brain.

Besides the demand in glucose, which is high at the end of foetal life, we must once more recall the importance of the demand in iodine, since this mineral is essential for thyroid hormone production and since thyroid hormones are needed for brain development. We must keep in mind that iodine deficiency is the most common nutritional deficiency among humans and that there are significant alterations of the levels of thyroid hormones during pre-eclampsia–eclampsia.

Since the brain is an eminently fatty organ, we'll focus on lipids. The concept of maternal–foetal conflicts suggests we should establish a new classification of the numerous well-documented biological imbalances related to the metabolism of fatty acids.[10]

(The end of this subchapter about "interspecies comparisons of maternal foetal conflicts" may be skimmed through by those who are not familiar with the language of biochemists and the language of the medical profession.)

We must keep in mind that in this specifically human pregnancy disease the level of the "brain specific fatty acid" remains stable. This specific fatty acid, commonly called DHA, is the longest and most desaturated molecule of fatty acid; it belongs to the omega-3 family. Maintaining stable DHA levels has an enormous cost: the level of the parent molecule EPA is about 10 times lower than in normal pregnancy.[11] These are exactly the data we should expect when assuming that brain development is a priority among humans.

Significant concordant data leads to the conclusion that when the amount of omega-3 available is low, the first compensatory effect is a collapse in the level of the previous molecule in the metabolic pathway (EPA). This precipitating factor explains the well-known imbalances in the system of prostaglandins. Such interpretations are supported by the Curacao study, which looked at the fatty acid composition of maternal and umbilical cord platelets.[12] The use of biomarkers of dietary intake of lipids has demonstrated that a diet poor in omega-3 fatty acids is a risk factor for pre-eclampsia. Studies of the red cell fatty acid profile found that women with the lowest levels of omega-3 fatty acids were 7.6 times more likely to have had their pregnancies complicated by preeclampsia compared with those women with the highest levels.[13]

If we view the well-documented metabolic imbalances in that way it is understood that many kinds of factors can modify the expression of maternal–foetal conflict. The point of departure for studies of the specifically human pregnancy disease should not be a theoretical framework focusing on faulty placentation. It should be the prevalence of the real disease multiplied by one hundred in some human groups compared with others, independently of what modern medical practices can offer.

Such perspectives would shed new light on some puzzling aspects of the disease:

- The fact that there is a significant association between pre-eclampsia and high birth weight babies, in addition to the well-known association with small-for-gestational-age fetuses.[14]
- The association of pre-eclampsia with lower infant mortality in preterm babies.[15]
- The reported association of pre-eclampsia with a reduced risk of cerebral palsy.[16]
- The fact that eclampsia is more frequent in the case of multiple pregnancies.
- The fact that 5 to 15 years after pre-eclampsia, women have brain alterations that cannot be explained by their cardiovascular profile.[17] This suggests that pregnant women who have difficulty meeting the specific nutritional needs of the developing brain of their unborn babies also have difficulty meeting the nutritional needs of their own brain.
- The fact that eclampsia is principally a disease of first pregnancy leads to recall that the metabolism of omega-3 fatty acids is influenced by parity.[18] The capacity to synthetise DHA is depleted with repeated pregnancies. It is as if brain development is a higher priority in the case of a first baby. It is also significant that the capacity to synthetise DHA is severely constrained in post-menopausal women and men. It is as if, among women in the reproductive phase of their life, the capacity to feed a developing brain is essential.[19–21]

In an enlarged theoretical context, it is becoming easy to interpret unexpected effects of some new medical strategies. This is the case of a reduced risk of preeclampsia after treatment of gestational diabetes by hypoglycaemic agents, such as metformin, which is transferred to the foetus through the placenta, and insulin.[22] Let us recall that the foetal developing brain is consuming huge amounts of glucose. The placenta, as the "advocate of the baby", tends to manipulate maternal physiology to satisfy such needs. Some pregnant women, particularly those who belong to a particular metabolic type, must make a bigger effort than others. A supplement of glucose given to such women is followed by an immediate high peak of glycaemia. This is the principle of the "glucose tolerance test". "Gestational diabetes" is not a disease: it is the interpretation of a test. It is easy to understand that in the case of a macrosomia (high weight foetus), the demand is high and not easily satisfied. In general, the label gestational diabetes should simply lead to recommendations in terms of lifestyle (nutrition and physical activity).

There are reasons to be critical about the active pharmacological treatment of gestational diabetes. One of the effects of medications such as metformin or insulin given to the mother is to reduce the amount of glucose crossing the placenta and therefore to moderate foetal weight and to hinder brain development. Medical treatment is neutralising the message expressed by the placenta as an endocrine gland. If foetal brain development is hindered, the demand in "brain selective nutrients" and therefore the risks of pre-eclampsia are reduced. Many practitioners may be satisfied to moderate birth weight and to reduce the risks of pre-eclampsia. Those who consider brain development as a priority among humans may have different points of view.

An enlarged theoretical context associated with a renewed interest in real eclampsia would lead to greater importance of what we can learn from brain imaging techniques. One of the most valuable published studies so far was performed in India.[23] One hundred and four consecutive women with eclampsia were subjected to magnetic resonance imaging (MRI). In this particular study the objective was to identify predictors of "posterior encephalopathy syndrome". We must save from oblivion an American study dated 1993 comparing 16 cases of severe preeclampsia and 10 cases of real eclampsia: there are specific changes in real eclampsia only.[24]

Of course, the ulterior motive is the advent of new generations of therapeutic strategies that could not easily emerge as long as the topics of interest were dominated by placental implantation. For example, starting from theoretical considerations, it has been suggested that an emulsion of lipid for intravenous use ("intralipids") might provide essential fatty acids in situations of emergency and be brain protective in the case of severe pre-eclampsia.[25] It is also possible that therapeutic strategies already in use in a great diversity of medical disciplines will unexpectedly inspire new emergency treatments of severe preeclampsia and eclampsia. This might be the case, for example, of the association (already used in periodontology) of aspirin and the fatty acid DHA.[26] It would make sense, theoretically, to consider such an association to treat also severe pre-eclampsia.

Our interdisciplinary overview of "the disease of theories" is leading us to challenge an old assumption and to raise a new question: is eclampsia first and foremost a disease of the agricultural phase of human history?

We must keep in mind that from the advent of agriculture until recently the diet of human beings has been cereal based. Maize was first domesticated by indigenous peoples in southern Mexico about 10,000 years ago before becoming a staple food in many parts of the world. Rice has been widely consumed, particularly in Asia: it is the symbol of the Chinese culture. In the Middle East and Europe, the word "bread" has been synonymous with "food". To refer to their basic needs, the Romans were using the phrase "panem and circenses", which literally means "bread and circuses". The word "bread" has the same enlarged meaning in Holy Scriptures.

To provide preliminary answers to this crucial question, we would need documents about the prevalence of eclampsia in Palaeolithic societies. It is notable that neither Daniel Everett, who spent several decades among an Amazonian pre-Neolithic ethnic group, nor Marjorie Shostak and Melvin Konner, who wrote about childbirth among the African hunter–gatherers the !Kung San, nor Wulf Schiefenhovel, who provided documents among the Eipos, in New Guinea, ever mentioned one case of eclampsia, although it is an easy to diagnose disease. The skeleton of a 20-year-old woman buried with a baby in her womb estimated at 8 months gestation was found near the Southern Italian Adriatic coast. It might have been a case of eclampsia fromabout 28,000 years ago. In fact, the cause of the deaths is unknown.[28]

References

1. Knight M (2007) Eclampsia in the United Kingdom 2005. *BJOG* **114(9)**:1072–78.
2. Watanabe K, Suzuki Y and Yamamoto T (2013) Incidence of eclampsia in Japanese women. *Hypertens Pregnancy* **1(1)**:31–4.
3. Begum MR, Begum A, Quadir E, *et al.* (2004) Eclampsia: Still a problem in Bangladesh. *MedGenMed* **6(4)**:52.
4. Ouattara A, Ouédraogo CMR, Ouédraogo A, *et al.* (2015) Eclampsia at the University hospital Yalgado of Ouagadougou (Burgina Faso) from 1 April 2013 to 31 March 2014. *Bulletin de la Société Exotique* **108(5)**:316–23.
5. (1912) *Hommage au Professeur Pinard, 13 novembre 1910.* G Steinheil publisher, Paris.
6. Ross RA (1947) Late toxemias of pregnancy: the number one obstetrical problem in the South. *Am J Obstet Gynecol* **54(5)**:723–30.
7. Ferguson JH (1951) Maternal death in the rural South: a study of forty-seven consecutive cases. *JAMA* **146**:1388.
8. Hamlin RH (1952) The prevention of eclampsia and pre-eclampsia. *Lancet* **1(6698)**:64–8.
9. Brewer GS, Brewer T. *What Every Pregnant Woman Should Know.* Random House, New York.
10. Odent M (2000) Pre-eclampsia as a maternal — fetal conflict. The link with fetal brain development. *International Society for the Study of Fatty Acids and Lipids (ISSFAL) News* **7**:7–10.

11. Wang Y, Kay HH and Killam AP (1991) Decreased levels of polyunsaturated fatty acids in pre-eclampsia. *Am J Obstet Gynecol* **164**:812–8.

12. Velzing-Aarts FV, van der Klis FR, van der Dijs FP and Muskiet FA (1999) Umbilical vessels of preeclamptic women have low contents of both n-3 and n-6 long-chain polyunsaturated fatty acids. *Am J Clin Nutr* **69**:293–8.

13. Williams MA, Zingheim RW, King IB and Zebelman AM (1995) Omega-3 fatty acids in maternal erythrocytes and risk of pre-eclampsia. *Epidemiology* **6**:232–7.

14. Xiong X, Demianczuk NN, Buekens P and Saunders LD (2000) Association of preeclampsia with high birth weight for age. *Am J Obstet Gynecol* **183**:148–55.

15. Chen XK, Wen SW, Smith G, *et al.* (2006) Pregnancy-induced hypertension is associated with lower infant mortality in preterm singletons. *BJOG* **113**:544–51.

16. Murphy DJ, Sellers S, MacKenzie IZ, *et al.* (1995) Case-control study of antenatal and intrapartum risk factors for cerebral palsy in very preterm singleton babies. *Lancet* **346**:1449–54.

17. Siepmann T, Boardman H, Bilderbeck A, *et al.* (2017) Long-term cerebral white and gray matter changes after preeclampsia. *Neurology* **88(13)**:1256–64. doi: 10.1212/WNL.0000000000003765.

18. Carlson E and Salem N (1991) Essentiality of omega-3 fatty acids in growth and development in infants. In: Simopoulos AP, Kifer RR, Martin RE and Barlow SM (eds.) *Effects of Polyunsaturated Fatty Acids in Seafoods. World Rev Nutr Diet* **66**:74–86. Karger, Basel.

19. Lohner S, Fekele K, Marosvölgyi T and Decsi T (2013) Gender differences in the long-chain polyunsaturated fatty acid status: systematic review of 51 publications. *Ann Nutr Metab* **62(2)**:98–112. doi: 10.1159/000345599.

20. Burdge G (2004) Alpha-linolenic acid metabolism in men and women: nutritional and biological implications. *Curr Opin Clin Metan Care* **7(2)**:137–44.

21. Burdge GC and Wootton SA (2002) Conversion of alpha-linolenic acid to eicosapentaenoic, docosapentaenoic and docosahexaenoic acids in young women. *Br J Nutr* **88(4)**:411–20.

22. Barbour LA, Scifres C, Valent AM, *et al.* (2018) A cautionary response to SMFM statement: pharmacological treatment of gestational diabetes. *Am J Obstet Gynecol* **219(4)**:367.e1–367.e7. doi: 10.1016/j.ajog.2018.06.013.

23. Verma AK, Gang RK, Pradeep Y, *et al.* (2017) Posterior encephalopathy syndrome in women with eclampsia: Predictors and outcome. *Pregnancy Hypertens* **10**:74–82. doi: 10.1016/j.preghy.2017.06.004.

24. Digre KB, Varner MW, Osborn AG and Crawford S (1993) Cranial magnetic resonance imaging in severe preeclampsia vs eclampsia. *Arch Neurol* **50(4)**:399–406.

25. Joseph Eldor and Stark M (2018) Intralipid treatment of preeclampsia/eclampsia? *J Health Sci Dev* **1(1)**: 48–60.

26. El-Sharkawi H, Aboelsaad N and Eliwa M (2010) Adjunctive treatment of chronic periodontitis with daily dietary supplementation with omega-3 fatty acids and low-dose aspirin. *J Peridontol* **81(11)**:1635–43. doi: 10.1902/jop.2010.090628.

27. McGinnis R, Steinthorsdottir V, Williams NO, *et al.* (2017) Variants in the fetal genome near FLT1 are associated with risk of preeclampsia. *Nat Genet* **49(8)**:1255–60. doi: 10.1038/ng.3895.

28. Robillard PY, Scioscia M, Coppola D, *et al.* (2018) La "Donna di Ostuni", a case of eclampsia 28,000 years ago? *J Matern Fetal Neonatal Med* **31(10)**:1381–84. doi: 10.1080/14767058.2017.1312333.

Homo Navigator

Abstract

Many islands and coastal areas of the Palaeolithic period are now immersed as an effect of significant fluctuations of sea levels. This may explain a tendency to underestimate the proportion of humans who were living on the land–sea interface before the "Neolithic revolution", since their fossils will never be easily found. It is to a great extent by seafaring that our ancestors populated the planet. At a time when a new understanding of human nature cannot be ignored, and after raising questions inspired by the prevalence of pathological conditions, such as eclampsia, it appears necessary to synthesise available data about "Homo navigator". We provide reasons to focus on the colonisation of the Mediterranean basin and the Pacific Rim. We also provide reasons to raise questions about the mysterious spatial skills of long-distance migrants, whether they are birds or humans.

Two Basic Kinds of Palaeolithic Lifestyle

These questions about Palaeolithic societies are crucial at a time when we dare to present Homo as "the marine chimpanzee" since, when a trait is apparently specific to our species, we must look at what we have in common with mammals adapted to the sea or coastal areas.[1,2] Until now "Palaeolithic Homo" was almost synonymous with hunter–gatherer. There have been countless documents and speculations about the diet of hunter–gatherers. The term "paleo diet" is now commonly used in daily conversation.

Today, we must also raise questions about the lifestyle of "Homo navigator". It is to a great extent as navigators that our ancestors colonised the planet, particularly the Mediterranean basin and the Pacific Rim. To refer concomitantly to the lifestyles, particularly the diet, of "Homo agricultural" and of "Homo navigator" is a way to realise the extraordinary dietary flexibility of members of our species.

It is established that many islands and coastal areas of the Palaeolithic eras are now immersed as an effect of significant fluctuations of sea levels. This may explain a tendency to underestimate the proportion of humans who were living in coastal areas, since their fossils will never be easily found. However, we must mention that the skull of a Neanderthal, dated about 40,000 years old, has been found at the bottom of the Northern sea, about 16 km from the Dutch coast. Britain used to be a peninsula of Europe: the sea level was about 120 metres lower during the period of glaciation that ended about 18,000 years ago.

The Mediterranean Basin

Where the Mediterranean Basin is concerned, there is evidence that middle Palaeolithic humans (300,000 to 30,000 years ago) were living in both the Moroccan part of North Africa and in the Iberian Peninsula. Even when the sea levels were as low as possible, only navigators could cross the Strait of Gibraltar.

On the African side, significant hominin fossils have been found, in particular at Jebel Irhoud, an archaeological site close to Marrakech.[3] In 2017, following new digs and tests using advanced techniques, the remains were reanalysed. It appeared that they belonged to a big brained Homo and that they were about 300,000 years old. The findings had been initially interpreted as Neanderthals. After that they have been interpreted as Sapiens or a population of Sapiens that had interbred with Neanderthals.[4] On the Iberian side, the most significant documents were found in Vanguard and Gorham's Caves, that lie on the Eastern side of Gibraltar. These Palaeolithic humans, classified as Neanderthals, exploited seals, dolphins and fish. They were undoubtedly navigators.[5]

Convincing evidence regarding the seafaring ability of Mediterranean hominins comes originally from Sicily, Sardinia and Cyprus. It is almost established that the Neanderthal variety of big brained Homo could reach Mediterranean islands by canoeing.[6-9] Their distinctive "Mousterian" stone tools are found on the Greek mainland and, intriguingly, have also been found on the Greek islands of Lefkada and Kefalonia. According to George Ferentinos, from the University of Patras, Greece, the sea would have been at least 180 metres deep when Neanderthals were in the region. Let us add that, in 2008, Thomas Strasser, from Providence College in Rhode Island, found similar stone tools on Crete, which he says are at least 130,000 years old. Crete has been an island for some 5 million years and is 40 kilometres from its closest neighbour. There is food for thought in the comments by Thomas Strasser: "Early hominids may have used the seas as a highway, rather than seeing them as a barrier".

The Pacific Rim

Where the colonisation of the Pacific Rim is concerned, we are also reaching radically new ways of thinking.

We must first keep in mind that hominid remains and stone tools dating back 700,000 to 800,000 years ago have been found on Flores Island, Indonesia, by the joint Australian–Indonesian research team headed by Michael Morwood. According to Morwood, the mysterious Homo floresiensis got there by using boats.[10] We must also mention that the remains of another hominin have been found in the island of Luzon, 3000 km from Flores. The discoveries of "Homo floresiensis" and "Homo luzonensis" might intensify the hunt for more extinct hominins in this part of the world and help phrasing new questions about the relationship between Hominins and the sea.

The most undisputable evidence for the first use of boats in the South Pacific region is the human migration from Sundaland to the ancient continent of Sahul (which is now divided into the Australian mainland, New Guinea and Tasmania), more than 50,000 years ago. Given that this migration required navigating a 970 km long band of islands and at least 10 ocean straights, it seems likely that boats and coastal navigation existed for at least some time before that.

Let us recall that one of the cradles of human civilisation has been the prehistorical lowlands of the Southeast Asian peninsula. This area, commonly called the "Sundaland", was above sea level during the last ice age. It was twice the size of India, and included what we now call Indo-China, Malaysia and Indonesia. From there, while some of our ancestors migrated towards the South, others migrated towards the North, reaching the Japanese Archipelago, also about 40,000 years ago.

As for the migrations towards the American continents, the sudden need to re-write their history justifies, more than ever, the concept of "Homo navigator". The comparative importance of migrations along the coasts has probably been underestimated in the past.

Until recently, according to theories based on archaeological data, the ancestors of the indigenous cultures of the American continents had appeared in what is now New Mexico, where they developed the "Clovis culture". They were supposed to have reached the North American continent through an ice-free corridor that extended from Alaska to Montana. We have recently learned that life came to the ice-free Canadian corridor too late to sustain this theory.

It is undisputable now that there has been a more diverse set of founding populations of the continent than previously accepted.[11,12] Complex streams of gene flow between North and South America have been previously unappreciated. Comments published in *Nature* summarise the current situation: "Ancient genomics paints a messy picture of America's first settlers".

The implications of recent findings are enormous. Questions about the "Australasia genetic signal" even suggest that the wacky and even apparently absurd hypothesis of a human migration towards the coasts of South America via the Southern part of the Pacific Ocean should not be radically dismissed. We must keep in mind that 20,000 years ago, when the sea levels were more than 100 metres lower than today, there were countless Islands in the Southern Pacific Ocean. Some of them still exist: Pitcairn Islands, Easter Island, Sala y Gomez, Desventuradas Islands, San Felix, San Ambrosio, Alejandro Selkirk and Robinson Crusoe, in particular. We must also keep in mind what is known about how early navigators were guided in unchartered seas and the important part played by birds.[13] It is significant that the Rapa Nui name for Sala y Gomez island means "Bird's islet on the way to Hiva". The strong spatial skills of birds such as the terns remain mysterious. Even in historical times, explorers were still guided by birds. Vincente Pinzón, the Spanish navigator who sailed with Christopher Columbus on their first voyage to the New World, was quoted as saying: "Those birds know their business". Is it plausible that archaic navigators had reached the highly productive ecosystem related to the Humboldt current, which runs along the South American coast? Still about the Pacific area, we must keep in mind that the Marshall Islands, that lie more than 2000 miles from the nearest continent, have been discovered and colonised about

3,000 years ago by seafarers from South East Asia who were relying on the art of "wave piloting". Wave pilots steer by the feeling of the ocean itself: before the age of stick charts, they could perceive disruptions in ocean swells by islands. It is probable that ancestral humans have also used a combination of wind and stars to navigate. We may be amazed by the capacity of Homo navigator to plan extremely daring voyages. Such audacious behaviours can be explained by a conception of the world according to which the ocean is full of islands.

We have the proof that the canoe squadrons of archaic Homo were carrying men and women since, after reaching new territories, they could reproduce and start off populations. This fact can inspire questions about gender differences at a time when the concept of male superiority in spatial thinking is challenged.[14,15] It seems more appropriate today to think in terms of advantageous complementarity between male and female brain functions.

It is still premature to evaluate the real importance of reported findings at the Cerutti Mastodon site in South California.[16] According to the authors of the investigations, there is evidence that, 130,000 years ago, an unidentified variety of Homo was living there. These humans were apparently endowed with sufficient manual dexterity and experiential knowledge to use hammerstones and anvils. Critics have claimed that alternative interpretations have not been ruled out.[17] We must keep in mind, on the other hand, the point of view of the archaeologist Ruth Gruhn. Her examination of the broken bone fragments in the Cerutti Mastodon Site collection indicates that the hypothesis of breakage by modern heavy machinery is invalid, as a thick precipitate of soil carbonate on the broken surfaces proves that the breakage was very ancient.[18]

Such considerations about Homo navigator, as one of the prototypes of pre-historic Homo, should renew our curiosity about the nature of Homo and the limits of human adaptability.

References

1. Odent M (2017) *The Birth of Homo, the Marine Chimpanzee.* Pinter & Martin, London.
2. Odent M (1996) Are we marine chimps? In: Beech BL (ed.) *Water Birth Unplugged.* Books for Midwives Press.
3. Callaway E (2017) Oldest Homo sapiens fossil claim rewrites our species history. *Nature News, 8 June 2017.* doi: 10.1038/nature.2017.22114.
4. Hublin JJ, Ben-Ncer A, Bailey SE, *et al.* (2017) New fossils from Jebel Irhoud, Morocco and the pan-African origin of Homo sapiens. *Nature* **546(7657)**:289–92. doi: 10.1038/nature22336.
5. Stringer CB, Finlayson JC, Barton RNE, *et al.* (2008) Neanderthal exploitation of marine mammals in Gibraltar. *Proc Natl Acad Sci USA* **105(38)**:14319–24. doi: 10.1073/pnas.0805474105.
6. Yirka B (1 March 2012) Evidence suggests Neanderthals took to boats before modern humans. *phys.org news.* Available at: https://phys.org/news/2012-03-evidence-neanderthals-boats-modern-humans.html. Accessed 5 May 2016.
7. Marshall M (29 February 2012) Neanderthals were very ancient mariners *New Scientist.* Available at: https://www.newscientist.com/article/mg21328544-800-neanderthals-were-ancient-mariners/. Accessed 5 May 2016.
8. Choi CQ (15 November 2012) Ancient Mariners: Did Neanderthals sail to Mediterranean islands? *LiveScience.* Available at: https://www.livescience.com/24810-neanderthals-sailed-mediterranean.html. Accessed 5 May 2016.
9. Ferentinos G, Gkioni M, Geraga M and Papatheodorou G (2012) Early seafaring activity in the southern Ionian Islands, Mediterranean Sea. *J Archaeol Sci* **39**:2167–76.
10. Morwood MJ, Van Oosterzee P (2007) *A New Human: The Startling Discovery and Strange Story of the "Hobbits" of Flores, Indonesia.* Smithsonian Books, Washington DC.
11. Moreno-Mayar JV, Vinner L, de Barros Damgaard P, *et al.* (2018) Early human dispersals within the Americas. *Science* **362(6419)**:eaav2621. doi: 10.1126/science.aav2621.

12. Posth C, Nakatsuka N, Lazaridis I, *et al.* (2018) Reconstructing the deep population history of Central and South America. *Cell* **175(5)**:1185–1197.e22. doi.org/10.1016/j.cell. 2018.10.027.

13. Hornell J (1946) The role of birds in early navigation. *Antiquity* **20(79)**: 142–9. dx.doi.org/10.1017/S0003598X0001953031.

14. Jones CM, Braithewaite VA, Healy SD (2003) The evolution of sex differences in spatial ability. *Behav Neurosci* **117**(3): 403–11

15. Clint EK, Sober E, *et al.* (2012). Male superiority in spatial navigation: adaptation or side effect? *Q REV Biol* **87**(4): 289–313.

16. Holen SR, Deméré TA, Fisher DC *et al.* (2017) A 130,000-year-old archaeological site in southern California, USA. *Nature* **544**: 479–83. doi: 10.1038/nature22065.

17. Ferraro JV, Binetti KM, Weist LA, *et al.* (2018) Contesting early archaeology in California. *Nature* **554(7691)**: E1–E2.

18. Gruhn R (2018) Observations concerning the Cerutti Mastodon Site. *PaleoAmerica* **4(2)**:101–2. doi.org/10.1080/20555563.2018.1467192.

9 The Blind Men and the Elephant

Abstract

After providing reasons to conjecture that what happens during the phase of birth preparation might have lifelong consequences, we must emphasise the need for a new generation of epidemiological studies. This need appears clearly when looking at the contents of the "Primal Health Research Database". Since 1986, we have been collecting published epidemiological studies that explore correlations between "the primal period" and what happens later on in life in terms of health and personality trait (www.primalhealthresearch.com). The "primal period" starts at conception and is over around the first birthday. It may be presented as the phase of life when our basic adaptive systems — those involved in what we commonly call health — are reaching a high degree of maturity. The point is that, according to the phase of history and the background of those who explore the database, there is a tendency to focus on one of the three components of the primal period (foetal life, the birth itself, or the year following birth) and to ignore the periods of transition, including the phase of birth preparation.

For thousands of years, the parable of the blind men exploring an elephant has inspired comments, passionate discussions and theories. Each blind man, after touching one part of the elephant's body tended to project his partial experience as the whole truth. Who was as close as possible to the truth? The one saying "it is like a rope" after touching the tail? The one saying "it is like a thick branch of a tree" after touching the trunk? The one saying "it is like a big hand fan" after touching an ear? The one saying "it is like a huge wall" after touching the belly? The one saying "it is like a solid pipe" after touching the tusk? I'll suggest that the one who would have explored a connection between two big parts of the body (a major articulation) would have had an advantage compared with all the others.

The Specialised Explorers of the Primal Health Research Database

I cannot help thinking of this parable when considering comments inspired by the contents of the "Primal Health Research database". Since 1986, in our database, we have been collecting published epidemiological studies that explore correlations between "the primal period" and what happens later on in life in terms of health and personality trait (www.primalhealthresearch.com). The "primal period" starts at conception and is over around the first birthday. It may be presented as the phase of life when our basic adaptive systems — those involved in what we commonly call health — are reaching a high degree of maturity. The point is that, according to the phase of history and the background of those who explore the database, there is a tendency to focus on one of the three components of the primal period (foetal life, the birth itself, or the year following birth) and to ignore the periods of transition.

In the 1990s, the "foetal origins of disease hypothesis" was inspired by the countless studies published by the "Barker group", a team of British epidemiologists based in Southampton. According to this hypothesis, reduced foetal growth is associated with chronic conditions later on in life. An increased susceptibility results from adaptation made by the foetus in an environment limited in its supply of nutrients. An exploration of our database through keywords such as "coronary heart disease", "stroke", "diabetes" or "hypertension" gives access to data that have attracted the attention of academic medical circles.

In spite of the small number of valuable relevant epidemiological studies available in our database, we must mention the current strong curiosity in the possible effects of foetal exposure to a great diversity of factors associated with modern lifestyle, including the possible side effects of medication used during pregnancy, such as valproate. There are still unanswered questions about "hormonal disruptors", particularly substances that mimic oestrogens, such as Bisphenol A (from plastics and epoxy resins), polychlorinated biphenyls (from flame retardants and plasticisers) and phthalates (plasticisers and personal care products). There are still many questions about ionising radiations. The most valuable epidemiological studies are about long-term effects on brain development and cognitive functions of prenatal exposure to air pollution (polycyclic aromatic hydrocarbons) and effects on lung functions of prenatal exposure to fine particulate matter.[1-3]

Since the database was put into service, the continuous interest in the possible long-term consequences of what happens during the year following birth has been dominated by questions related to different modes of infant feeding. We must keep in mind that the advent of modern epidemiology — particularly primal health research — has been preceded by a phase of history when breastfeeding was devalued: the concept of "humanised milk" had been instrumental in the popularisation of bottle feeding. The creation of La Leche League by seven mothers, in 1956, may be interpreted as the symbol of an emerging new awareness: the objective was to transmit an understanding of breastfeeding as an important element in the healthy development of the child. It is significant that, over the years, the keyword "breastfeeding" offered by our database has remained highly productive. There is a strong interest for this family of studies among groups encouraging breastfeeding.

By comparison, it appears that our database has rarely been explored through the keyword "vaccination", although there are valuable huge studies (particularly from Denmark) inspired by this topic. We must emphasise that, in general, epidemiologists have never detected long term non-specific effects on health of any kind of infancy vaccinations. Such detections are difficult since, apart from BCG, infancy vaccinations have never been evaluated through randomised controlled trials. The point is that, in this field, the media, the general public and even health professionals share a tendency to be guided by opinions, passionate points of view and theories rather than hard data. In our database, on the other hand, we collect only studies exploring correlations and we avoid focusing on hypotheses regarding possible cause and effect relationship.

Taboo-Induced Blindness

The attitudes regarding epidemiological studies related to the birth process are intriguing. Until the end of the 20th century, there was a mysterious cultural lack of interest in the possible long-term consequences of the way babies are born. In fact, it was more than a lack of curiosity. It is as if, until recently, introducing such a topic was breaking a taboo. Those who dared to break the taboo were, one way or another, more or less neutralised.

One of the most typical examples is the case of Otto Rank, who had been working closely with Sigmund Freud and had often been considered his most brilliant disciple. The turning point was in 1924, when Rank dared to publish *Das Trauma der Geburt* (The trauma of Birth), exploring how art, myths, religion, philosophy and therapy were illuminated by the period of transition between intra-uterine and extra-uterine life. After the publication of such a book, Rank was eliminated from the Vienna Psychoanalytic Society.

Still in the context of the first half of the 20th century, the case of Maria Montessori is different. The part of her work about school age children is universally known and has been highly influential. It is only what she wrote about childbirth that has been electively neutralised. It is possible to read the most detailed of her numerous biographies in a great variety of languages without having a clue of the importance she gave to the way babies are born. This is the beginning of the chapter about "The newborn child" in her book entitled "The Secret of Childhood", (which is an adaptation to the English language of a book originally published in French in 1930): "At birth a child does not enter into a natural environment but into one that has already been extensively modified by men. It is an alien environment that has been built up at nature's expense by men...At no other period of his life does a man experience such a violent conflict and struggle, and consequent suffering, as at the time of birth. This is a period that certainly deserves to be seriously studied, but as yet no such study has been made..." It is as if Maria Montessori was already anticipating the branch of epidemiology we call "Primal Health Research".

After referring to this powerful deep-rooted taboo, it is easy to interpret the paucity, before the turn of the century, of epidemiological studies focusing on the birth itself. This paucity is associated with a cultural lack of curiosity that can be illustrated through examples, such as the "Dunedin study". This is a longitudinal study of 1,037 people born in the same hospital in Dunedin, New Zealand, between 1st April 1975 and 31st March 1976. The participants were regularly assessed a dozen times between age 3 and age 45. This study inspired hundreds of papers about many aspects of health and behaviour. It is significant that none of these studies took into account the modes of birth. This should have been possible since all participants were born in the same hospital in the mid-1970s.

However, we must mention that keywords such as forceps delivery, ventouse (or vacuum) and caesarean had already started to be occasionally productive several decades ago. It is worth saving from oblivion some of the oldest entries included in our database. We must mention, in particular, an evaluation of the intelligence quotient (IQ) scores of 97 American school children born in the same hospital in the years 1952–1954 by caesarean section after prolonged labour. After considering the IQ of the other members of the families, it appeared that a trial of labour exceeding 12 hours had detrimental effects.[4] This study has in retrospect an irreplaceable value, since it preceded the use of drips of synthetic oxytocin, a factor that might independently influence brain development. Today, it provides food for thought at a time when the capacity to give birth is undoubtedly deteriorating. In the age of easy, fast and safe techniques of caesareans, it provides reasons, from the foetal point of view, to avoid long and difficult labours.

Getting Out of the Epidemiological cul-de-sac

In 2000, I could not help expressing my impatience while waiting for an emerging curiosity about the possible long-term effects of how babies are born. This is how I introduced the concept of "cul-de-sac epidemiology".[5] In this framework I included research about topical issues. Despite the publication of this research in authoritative medical or scientific journals, the findings are shunned by the medical community and the media. "Cul-de-sac" epidemiological studies are not replicated and they are rarely quoted after publication.

The first example I offered to illustrate this concept was a series of convincing Swedish studies from the Karolinska Institute, published in the early 1990s. They led to the conclusion that certain obstetric medications, particularly opiates, are risk factors for the child to be drug addicted later on in life. My first innocent reaction, after meeting the authors of these studies, was that the media might spread the word and inspire comments at a time when drug addiction had become an important public health issue. I had imagined some clever journalists establishing a link between the "drug culture", that developed around 1970, and American births in the middle of the 20th century under the effect of a pharmacological cocktail including morphine ("twilight sleep").

It is highly significant that these Swedish studies remained ignored and were not replicated by other teams of researchers, so that the results have never been confirmed or invalidated. We must underline their great scientific value. They involved drug addicts born between 1945 and 1966. In a first report, the addicts were matched with their own siblings: the estimated relative risk was 4.7.[6] In a second report, two possible risk factors for drug addiction were weighed against each other: perinatal factors associated with obstetric medication and factors associated with socio-economic conditions.[7] In their last report, the authors considered the phenomenon of "contagious" transmission of drug addiction in certain residential area during adolescence.[8]

Of course, when considering these studies about drug addicts born in the middle of the 20th century, we must keep in mind that, at that time, morphine was commonly used in obstetrics and that nitrous oxide (the "laughing gas") was provided in higher concentrations than today. After the 1950s, synthetic opioid pain killers, such as pethidine (also known as meperidine or Demerol), have gradually replaced morphine. After the 1980s, when obstetrical anaesthesiology appeared as a new medical specialty, pethidine and epidural anaesthesia have been the dominant components of obstetrical analgesia. The point is that today, in a country such as the UK, about a third of labouring women receiving pethidine subsequently require an epidural, with an increased risk of instrumental delivery.

It is in such a context that a novel synthetic opioid — namely intravenous remifentanil — appears as having many advantages compared with pethidine. It has a very rapid onset and a short duration of action. The labouring woman is free to deliver boluses as needed ("patient controlled analgesia"). It has been demonstrated that after remifentanil, compared with pethidine, the proportion of epidurals is lower by half.[9]

Whatever the future of this new opioid, its advent is an opportunity to save from oblivion the Swedish studies and raise questions about the possible long-term effects of analgesics used in 21st century obstetrics. Until now only short-term effects have been considered. The main questions have been skipped. We must keep in mind that the placenta is effective at transferring opioids to the foetus. In the particular case of remifentanil, this has already been demonstrated with pregnant ewes.[10] Since, in this species, the placenta has a "synepitheliochorial" structure (several membranes between maternal and foetal blood streams) while the human placenta is "haemochorial" (only one membrane) it is quasi-certain that the human placenta is effective at transferring this novel analgesic drug. Randomised controlled trials starting now would provide valuable results within 20 years.

Another reason for my impatience, in 2000, was a study by Ryoko Hattori (Kumamoto, Japan). This study had remained ignored, although published in 1991 in an authoritative medical journal.[11] The main conclusion was clear: the "Kitasato University's method" of delivery is a risk factor for autism. This method is characterised by a planned delivery induced a week before the due date, plus sedative and analgesic agents. I considered this study so important that I found an opportunity to go to Kumamoto and meet Ryoko Hattori.

In the context of the 21st century, there has been a sudden accumulation of epidemiological studies related to the birth itself. Among the main topics we must mention autism, allergic diseases and auto immune diseases. One of the probable reasons for this new phenomenon is the strong interpretational value of emerging and fast-developing scientific disciplines such as epigenetics and modern bacteriology. There is a tendency to pay attention to correlations established by epidemiologists when the cause and effect relationship is made highly plausible. At the end of the 20th century the emergence of new scientific topics — such as the behavioural effects of oxytocin — already had the power to stimulate an interest in primal health research.

However, the taboo remains strong. Many review articles ignore epidemiological enquiries exploring risk factors during the period surrounding birth. For example, a "seminar" published in a highly authoritative medical journal about "autism spectrum disorder" was followed by 138 references.[12] Studies exploring risk factors during foetal life were reported. They included topics such as vaccination and influenza during pregnancy, folic acid intake, birthweight, serotonergic antidepressant and valproate. It is highly significant that none of the dozens of published studies looking at risk factors in the short period surrounding birth appeared on the list. Since we focus on the hours and days preceding birth, we find it important to know if obstetrical practices and aspects of modern lifestyle that interfere with this short period may have long term consequences. A 2017 synthesis of the results of valuable relevant studies concluded that both ways to shorten the period of "birth preparation" (pre-labour caesareans and induction) are associated with an increased risk of autism.[13]

There was a phase in the history of epidemiology when valuable studies regarding labour induction were not feasible. This was the case of countries where epidemiologists were using data provided by national birth registries. The concept of labour induction did not appear in Swedish and Danish registries until 1991.[14,15] This is why the first large authoritative study came from Australia.[16] This study had eliminated factors related the socio-economic and cultural context by comparing autistic children not only with controls, but also with siblings. Compared with their siblings, autistic children were more likely to have been induced. Compared with controls, they were more likely to be born after induction or by elective C-section. In all the relevant studies published after the Australian one, labour induction always appeared as a risk factor, in particular in the North Carolina study.[17] This study featured more than 600,000 live births linked with school records, including more than 5,500 autistic children. Compared with children born to mothers who received neither labour induction nor augmentation, children born to mothers who were induced and augmented, induced only, or augmented only experienced increased risks of autism after controlling for potential confounders related to socio-economic status, maternal health, pregnancy-related events and conditions, and birth year. The only discordant conclusions came from a Swedish study.[18] In this study, labour induction appeared as a significant risk factor, even after controlling for many confounding factors, but not after comparing with siblings.

On the day when the taboo induced blindness is overcome, the way will be open for a new generation of studies focusing on the modes of birth and their possible long-term consequences. For example, differences are commonly observed between genetically identical twins, although they spent their foetal life in the womb of the same mother and their infancy in the same environment. Researchers might consider that their births have often been different: for example, one twin had an easy birth, but not the other or one was born by the vaginal route and the other one by caesarean section.

Epidemiologists must overcome difficulties to dissociate the effects of the modes of birth and the effects of other particularities of modern lifestyle. They must take into account, for example, that we are at a turning point in the history of artificial light. All of us — including women during the phase of birth preparation — are highly exposed to the kind of light that inhibits melatonin release. This is why researchers might already be inspired by the results of animal experiments detecting a great diversity of negative long-term health outcomes on the offspring of maternal melatonin deprivation.[19]

Looking Towards the Future

After presenting "Primal Health Research" as a branch of epidemiology that has been in constant evolution since the 1980s, we are in a position to look towards the future. Let us recall that the advent of modern obstetrics during the second half of the 20th century had been mostly the effect of technological and technical advances, rather than scientific advances. There has been the "plastic revolution": it suddenly became safe to introduce plastic tubes in all organs of the body, including blood vessels and epidural space. There has been the electronic revolution: electronic foetal monitoring, in particular, has been widely used. There have been such advances in surgical and anaesthetic techniques that it became usual to perform a caesarean section in 20 minutes with minimal blood loss.

Today the main obstacles towards a necessary new awareness are taboo-induced blindness and overspecialisation. There is an increased need to focus on the frontiers between scientific disciplines. In other words, interdisciplinary approaches are more fruitful than pluridisciplinary perspectives. Let us keep in mind the advantages of the blind man who had access to a major articulation of the elephant body.[19]

References

1. Peterson BS, Rauh VA, Bansal R, et al. (2015) Effects of prenatal exposure to air pollutants (polycyclic aromatic hydrocarbons) on the development of brain white matter, cognition, and behavior in later childhood. *JAMA Psychiatry* **72(6)**:531–40. doi: 10.1001/jamapsychiatry.2015.57.

2. Jedrychowski WA and Perera FP (2015) Prenatal exposure to polycyclic aromatic hydrocarbons and cognitive dysfunction in children. *Environ Sci Pollut Res Int* **22(5)**:3631–9. doi: 10.1007/s11356-014-3627-8.

3. Jedrychowski WA and Perera FP (2010) Effect of prenatal exposure to fine particulate matter on ventilatory lung function of preschool children of non-smoking mothers. *Paediatr Perinat Epidemiol* **24(5)**:492–501. doi: 10.1111/j.1365-3016.2010.01136.x.

4. Roemer FJ, Rowland DY and Nuamah IF (1991) Retrospective study of fetal effects of prolonged labor before cesarean delivery. *Obstet Gynecol* **77(5)**:653–8.

5. Odent M (2000) Between circular and cul-de-sac epidemiology. *Lancet* **355**:1371.

6. Jacobson B, Nyberg K, Grönbladh L, *et al.* (1990) Opiate addiction in adult offspring through possible imprinting after obstetric treatment. *BMJ* **301**:1067–70.

7. Nyberg K, Allebeck P, Eklund G and Jacobson B (1992) Socio-economic versus obstetric risk factors for drug addiction in offspring. *Brit J Addict* **87**:1669–76.

8. Nyberg K, Allebeck P, Eklund G and Jacobson B (1993) Obstetric medication versus residential area as perinatal risk factors for subsequent adult drug addiction in offspring. *Paed and Perinatal Epid* **7**:23–32.

9. Wilson MJA, MacArthur C, Hewitt CA, *et al.* (2018) Intravenous remifentanil patient-controlled analgesia versus intramuscular pethidine for pain relief in labour (RESPITE): an open-label, multicentre, randomised controlled trial. *Lancet* **392(10148)**:662–72. doi: 10.1016/S0140-6736(18)31613-1.

10. Coonen JB, Marcus MA, Joosten EA, *et al.* (2010) Transplacental transfer of remifentanil in the pregnant ewe. *Br J Pharmacol* **161(7)**:1472–6.

11. Hattori R, Desimaru M, Nagayama I and Inoue K (1991) Autistic and developmental disorders after general anaesthetic delivery. *Lancet* **337(8753)**:1357–8. doi.org/10.1016/0140-6736(91)93045-B.

12. Lord C, Elsabbagh M and Baird G (2018) Seminar. Autism Spectrum Disorder. *Lancet* **392(10146)**:508–20. doi: 10.1016/S0140-6736(18)31129-2.

13. Wang C, Geng H, Liu W and Zhang G (2017) Prenatal, perinatal, and postnatal factors associated with autism: A meta-analysis. *Medicine (Baltimore)* **96(18)**:e6696. doi: 10.1097/MD.0000000000006696.

14. Hultman C, Sparen P and Cnattingius S (2002) Perinatal risk factors for infantile autism. *Epidemiology* **13**:417–23.

15. Larsson HJ, Eaton WW, Madsen KM, *et al.* (2005) Risk factors for autism: perinatal factors, parental psychiatric history, and socioeconomic status. *Am J Epidemiol* **161(10)**:916–25 (discussion 926–8).

16. Glasson EJ, Bower C, Petterson B, *et al.* (2004) Perinatal factors and the development of autism. *Arch Gen Psychiatry* **61**:618–27.

17. Gregory SG, Anthropolos R, Osgood CE, *et al*. (2013) Association of autism with induced or augmented childbirth in North Carolina Birth Record (1990–1998) and Education Research (1997–2007) databases. *JAMA Pediatr* **167(10)**:959–66. doi: 10.1001/jamapediatrics.2013.2904.

18. Oberg AS, D'Onofrio BM, Rickert ME, *et al*. (2016) Association of Labor Induction with Offspring Risk of Autism Spectrum Disorders. *JAMA Pediatr* **170(9)**:e160965. doi: 10.1001/jamapediatrics.2016.0965.

19. Motta-Teixeira LC, Machado-Nils AV, Battagello DS, *et al*. (2018) The absence of maternal pineal melatonin rhythm during pregnancy and lactation impairs offspring physical growth, neurodevelopment, and behavior. *Horm Behav* **105**:146–56. doi: 10.1016/j.yhbeh.2018.08.006.

Chapter

10 Sexual Orientation

Abstract

Since the epidemiological perspective appears necessary to evaluate the importance of the phase of birth preparation, we must wonder what kinds of studies are feasible in the foreseeable future. There are several reasons why we chose the issue of sexual orientation as an example. The first reason is that research tools have confirmed the importance of genetic factors: we therefore need to know about critical periods for gene–environment interaction. A second reason is that we will not have to wait many decades before identifying such personality traits as sexual orientation. We must also consider what is already known about the development of brain structures. For example, the end of foetal life is a phase of fast development of the hypothalamus and the structure of this part of the brain is not the same among heterosexual and homosexual men. The interpretation of relevant epidemiological studies will be facilitated if the common points and the differences between labour induction and pre-labour caesarean sections are simultaneously considered. These two medical interventions shorten the phase of birth preparation, but the first one is usually associated with prolonged pharmacological assistance while the second one is associated with stress deprivation. Whenever both of them appear correlated with the same pathological conditions or personality traits, the cause and effect relationship is highly plausible.

After analysing what we already know about the physiological reshaping that takes place in the phase of birth preparation, and after realising that our modern lifestyle has eliminated, shortened or dramatically altered this short phase of human life, the need for a new generation of epidemiological studies appears obvious. The critical period for gene–environment interaction is still imprecise for many kinds of states of health, pathological conditions and personality traits.

A Significant Example

We'll focus on the issue of sexual orientation as an example. For any study of the timing of gene–environment interaction, the first obligatory step is to refer to research tools that have confirmed and evaluated the importance of genetic factors. In general, twin and family studies offer useful points of departure.[1]

Twin and family tree studies are based on the principle that genetically-influenced traits run in families. The first modern study of patterns of homosexuality within families was published in 1985 by Richard Pillard and James Weinrich of Boston University. Since then, many other systematic studies of twins and siblings of gay men and lesbians have confirmed the initial results. The first pooled data for men showed that about 57% of identical twins, 24% of fraternal twins and 13% of brothers of gay men are also gay. For women, approximately 50% of identical twins, 16% of fraternal twins and 13% of sisters of lesbians are also lesbian. Michael Bailey, of North-western University, estimates that the overall heritability of sexual orientation is about 53% for men and 52% for women. One of the latest evaluations, based on the sexual orientation in a US national sample of twin and non-twin sibling pairs, confirmed that resemblance for sexual orientation was greater in the identical twins than in the fraternal twins and that sexual orientation is "substantially influenced by genetic factors."[2]

Family trees of male sexual orientation show that the rates of homosexuality in maternally-related males are far above the incidence of 2% in the average population, while the rates in paternal relatives are close to those of the average population. This finding raised the possibility of X chromosome involvement. Males have two sex chromosomes — Y inherited from the father and an X from the mother. Thus, a trait inherited through the mother's side logically might be influenced by a gene on one of her X chromosomes. This hypothesis is the basis of the X chromosome DNA analyses by Hamer and his colleagues. It appeared that one small area at the tip of the X chromosome — Xq28 — was shared by a large percentage of gay brothers.[3]

The results of such DNA analyses focusing on the X chromosome can help interpret a study among an Italian population, in which the mothers of gay men produced an average of 2.7 babies, compared to 2.3 for the other mothers.[4] It seems that maternally inherited factors favouring male homosexuality also promote female fecundity. This might explain why a genetic factor that reduces reproductive success remains in the population.

After recalling that sexual orientation is undoubtedly influenced by genetic factors, we must analyse the reasons why a new generation of epidemiological studies should consider the possible importance of the short phase of "birth preparation" as critical for gene–environment interaction.

One of the reasons is that the structure of the hypothalamus, which develops early in life, is not the same between heterosexual and homosexual men.

Simon LeVay, from the Salk Institute in San Diego, examined the hypothalamus of 41 subjects — 19 homosexual men who had died of complications of AIDS, 16 heterosexual men, and six heterosexual women. A characteristic feature of the brains of homosexual men is the small size of one hypothalamic nucleus, INAH 3, which LeVay found to be the same size as in women and only half the size found in heterosexual men.[5] INAH 3, he concludes, is dimorphic not with gender, but with sexual orientation. It is noticeable that six of the heterosexual men had died of AIDS but nevertheless had a large INAH 3.

Let us recall that, in the 1960s, Gunter Dorner had already conducted animal experiments in order to demonstrate the importance of the hypothalamus in sexual behaviour.[6-8] Dorner's conclusions were reinforced by Gorski and colleagues who found that, in rats, the size of the "sexually dimorphic nucleus" of the hypothalamus is established early in life and influences later sexual behaviour.[9] Subsequently, the same team of researchers showed that two nuclei of the hypothalamus, INAH 2 and 3, were twice as large in men as in women.[10]

The work of Gunter Dorner, from East Berlin, has undoubtedly generated a turning point in our understanding of the effect of environmental factors in sexual orientation.[10-12] Before Dorner there had been unsuccessful attempts to compare the hormonal profiles of adults expressing different sexual orientations. Dorner's studies revealed the importance of a critical period when the sexual differentiation of the brain happens.[13] While this critical period may vary slightly from one species to another, it is always around the time of birth.

Dorner started with animal experiments. Male rats were castrated on the first day of life and were injected with male hormones when adults. These male rats expressed a complete inversion of sexual behaviour. In other words, being deprived of testosterone during a critical period of sexual determination produced homosexual behaviour in their adult lives.

What we know now about the hormonal profile of homosexuals fits perfectly with the hypothesis of a transitory lack of testosterone during a critical period. Homosexuals usually have the same level of total testosterone as heterosexuals, but their level of "free testosterone" (testosterone that is not combined with other chemicals) is lower. The levels of pituitary hormones which control testicular functions are relatively high and so are the levels of oestrogens.

It is important to realise that if this hormonal profile were to be artificially reproduced in an adult, it would not give rise to homosexual behaviour. When a foetus is faced with a lack of testosterone at the end of pregnancy it compensates for this by increasing secretions of pituitary hormones. At the same time as the foetus tries to increase the level of male hormones by a feedback mechanism, it increases in parallel the level of oestrogens. In fact, oestrogens increase the binding capacity of sexual hormones with proteins and lower the level of free testosterone.

This raises the question of how and why some foetuses lack male hormones at the end of pregnancy. The answer could be that certain stressful situations at this time might trigger a high level of activity in the mother's adrenal glands. The adrenal glands release male hormones, the action of which is different from testosterone, but similar enough to compete with testosterone in the foetal brain to lower the amount of free testosterone.

At a time when we understand that the sexualisation of the brain takes place much later than the sexual differentiation of the genitals, we are in a position to phrase appropriate questions, such as: is there a critical period for the surge of testosterone that masculinises the foetal brain? Can prenatal stress, or other prenatal factors, play a causal role in human male sexual orientation?

To the first reasons why we have chosen the issue of sexual orientation to illustrate the need for a new generation of epidemiological studies, we must add another one, after recalling that the most powerful ways to interfere in the phase of physiological birth preparation (labour induction and pre-labour caesarean sections) were not common before the last decades of the 20th century. Epidemiological studies focusing on this particular issue should therefore be feasible without waiting, since a significant proportion of homosexual male humans are already sure and are not secretive about their sexual orientation in adolescence.

Furthermore, labour induction on the one hand, and pre-labour caesarean sections on the other hand, have their own associated factors. Labour induction is usually associated with prolonged phar-macological assistance, while pre-labour caesarean sections are associated with stress deprivation. If these two ways to shorten the phase of birth preparation are correlated with the same pathological conditions or personality traits, the cause and effect relationship is highly plausible. On the other hand, we'll have to wait several decades before identifying possible modern risk factors in early life for pathological conditions that express themselves late in life. We'll have to wait a still longer time before considering the issue of life expectancy.

Meanwhile

Meanwhile practitioners must keep in mind the results of published valuable studies involving men and women born before the advent of modern obstetrics. They must learn to think long term and to be cautious when interfering with the physiological processes. For example, the study demonstrating that men born from an eclamptic or pre-eclamptic mother have minimal risks of developing a prostate cancer involved boys born between 1874 and 1946.[14] The study demonstrating that the longer the time a boy has spent in the womb, the smaller the risks are of developing a prostate cancer in old age involved men born during the same period.[15] As for the study that demonstrated a markedly reduced risk of breast cancer in women whose mothers had eclampsia or pre-eclampsia, it involved girls born between 1874 and 1961.[16]

References

1. LeVay S and Hamer DH (1994) Evidence for a biological influence in male homosexuality. Sci Am 270(5):44–9.
2. Kendler KS, Thornton LM, Gilman SE and Kessler RC (2000) Sexual orientation in a U.S. national sample of twin and nontwin sibling pairs. Am J Psychiatry 157(11):1843–6.

3. Hamer DH, Hu S, Magnuson VL, *et al.* (1993) A linkage between markers on the X chromosome and male sexual orientation. *Science* **261**:321–7.

4. Corna F, Camperio-Ciani A and Capiluppi C (2004) Evidence for maternally inherited factors favouring male homosexuality and promoting female fecundity. *P R Soc B: Biol Sci* **271(1554)**:2217–21.

5. LeVay S (1991) A difference in hypothalamic structure between heterosexual and homosexual men. *Science* **253**:1034–7.

6. Dorner G and Staudt J (1968) Structural changes in the preoptic anterior hypothalamic area of the male rat, following neonatal castration and androgen substitution. *Neuroendocrinology* **3(3)**:136–40.

7. Dorner G and Staudt J (1969) Perinatal structural sex differentiation of the hypothalamus in rats. *Neuroendocrinol* **5**:103–6.

8. Dorner G and Staudt J (1969) Structural changes in the hypothalamic ventromedialnucleus of the male rat following neonatal castration and androgen treatment. *Neuroendocrinology* **4(4)**:278–81.

9. Gorski RA, Gordon JH, Shryne JE and Santham AM (1978) Evidence for a morphological difference within the medial preoptic area of the rat brain. *Brain Res* **148**:333–46.

10. Dorner G (1972) *Sexualhormonabhängige Gehirndifferenzierung und Sexualität*. Springer-Verlag, Vienna.

11. Dorner G (1976) *Hormones and Brain Differentiation*. Elsevier/North-Holland Biomedical Press, Amsterdam.

12. Dorner G (1977) Hormone dependent differentiation, maturation and function of the brain and sexual behavior. *Endokrinologie* **69**: 306–20.

13. Odent M (2008) Genesis of sexual orientation: From Plato to Dörner. *Hum Ontogen* **2(3)**:81–5. doi: 10.1002/huon.200800011.

14. Ekbom A, Wuu J, Adami HO, *et al.* (2000) Duration of gestation and prostate cancer risk in offspring. *Cancer Epidem Biomar* **9(2)**:221–3.

15. Ekbom A, Hsieh CC, Lipworth L, *et al.* (1996) Perinatal characteristics in relation to incidence of and mortality from prostate cancer *BMJ* **313(7053)**:337–41.

16. Ekbom A, Adami H-O, Hsieh CC, *et al.* (1997) Intrauterine environment and breast cancer risk, in women: a population-based study. *J Natl Cancer Inst* **89(1)**:71–6.

The Future of the Sorcerer's Apprentice

Abstract

After emphasising the need for a new generation of epidemiological studies and considering their feasibility, we must try to identify the priorities. It is possible if we bear in mind the mysterious turmoil regarding the comparative prevalence of many kinds of pathological conditions and personality traits among young generations born after the turning point in the history of childbirth. To illustrate the magnitude and the diversity of the questions that are suddenly emerging, we offer one example in the field of risk factors for well-defined frequent diseases (shingles), one example in the field of intellectual abilities (evolution of intellectual quotient) and one example related to "emotional health" (capacity for empathy). Meanwhile, one can imagine several scenarios. One of them would start with the sudden emergence of a new awareness leading to encourage cautious strategies before we know more. Another one would be to passively wait for hard data before reconsidering the dominant medical attitudes. If the second scenario prevails, there is a future for the sorcerer's apprentice.

A General Rule

While sexual orientation and cancers of glandular organs involved in human reproduction have already been seriously investigated in relation to the perinatal period among men and women born before the advent of modern obstetrics, we must now turn our attention to younger generations. There has been very recently a spectacular and mysterious turmoil regarding the comparative prevalence of many kinds of pathological conditions and personality traits. Interpretations are offered before being dismissed. As a general rule, theoreticians and researchers fail to consider the period surrounding birth. As long as the results of valuable epidemiological studies are not available, practitioners involved in childbirth are condemned to ignore the possible long-term consequences of early experiences or to follow their intuition. To illustrate the magnitude and the diversity of the questions that are suddenly emerging, we'll consider one example in the field of risk factors for well-defined frequent diseases, one example in the field of intellectual abilities and one example related to "emotional health".

Shingles

There are several reasons why we choose the example of shingles (or herpes zoster). The first reason is that this frequent viral disease is related to the immune status, an important aspect of health, strictly speaking. A second reason is that spectacular increases in the incidence of shingles have been reported in countries as diverse as the United States, Canada, the United Kingdom, Spain, Japan, Taiwan and Australia.[1-12] The most valuable sources of information are studies that have been possible in the particular case of the Olmsted County, in Minnesota, using precise data from 1945.[13,14] More than 8,000 cases were analysed. The prevalence of shingles increased from 0.76 per 1,000 person-year in 1945–1949 to 3.15 in 2000–2007. The rate of increase across the time was 2.5% per year. The prevalence of shingles significantly increased among all age groups and both sexes. The introduction of the varicella vaccination programme cannot explain the rate of increase. There have been unforeseen effects. One of them has been shortages in the recently introduced shingles vaccine as a result of high demand.

Let us recall that shingles results from reactivation of the varicella virus after a latency period. It is a painful eruptive disease often extending round the chest like a girdle (hence the name) or the face, particularly on the brow and round the eye. Risks of shingles increase with waning of immunity, which occurs with aging or immunosuppressive conditions or therapies.

Reasons for the increase remain mysterious. Some experts have theorised that adult exposure to children with chickenpox may provide a kind of protective booster effect against shingles. This booster effect has disappeared with the advent of chickenpox vaccination in the 1990s. This "external boosting" theory is now dismissed, because the rates of shingles had been increasing long before the chickenpox vaccine, because there has been no acceleration after the vaccine, and also because the same tendencies have been reported in countries where the use of chickenpox vaccine has never been widespread. It has also been emphasised that more and more young people are immunocompromised after undergoing organ transplants or surviving cancers. But this cannot explain the gradual rise in shingles dating back to the 1940s. The authors of the Minnesota study have also considered and dismissed theories linking the rise of shingles to climate change, agricultural pesticides, antibiotic resistance and stressful situations.

Our main comments are easily summarised: risk factors taking place in the period surrounding birth have not been taken into account until now, although the increased medicalisation of childbirth happened in parallel with the increased prevalence of shingles since World War II, and there are theoretical reasons to link these two phenomena.

Intellectual Quotient

How to explain that, among people born between World War II and the mid-1970s, the intellectual quotient had been gradually and significantly increasing, while it decreased among those born after 1975? That is how the question is usually phrased. We'll translate it into a more scientific language by referring to the "Flynn effect, its turning point, and its subsequent decline". The Flynn effect is the term commonly used in the academic literature to interpret the spectacular increase in population intelligence quotient observed throughout the 20th century.[15] The changes were fast, with measured intelligence typically increasing around three points per decade. However, in recent years, the Flynn effect has reversed in all countries where it has been seriously evaluated. How to interpret the current decline?[16]

One of the most valuable sources of reflection has used administrative register data with information on family relationships and intellectual ability for three decades of Norwegian male birth cohorts (conscripts).[17] It is notable that variations in intelligence scores inside families could be taken into account. This study has clearly established that the large decline in average intelligence quotients reflected environmental rather than genetic factors. Furthermore, it was possible to rule out several prominent hypotheses, particularly immigration and reduced education standards.

Once more we'll emphasise that factors taking place during the period surrounding birth, and particularly the phase of birth preparation, have not been taken into account. We cannot help recalling that it is precisely in the mid-1970s that the epidemic of labour induction became apparent. As early as 1975, there had been preliminary warnings about its possible long-term consequences, such as the BBC documentary film titled "A time to be born".[18] During the same decade, pre-labour caesarean sections became more common. It is notable that advances in techniques of artificial intelligence are more topical than the evolution of natural intelligence displayed by humans.

Capacity for Empathy

A high intellectual quotient and sophisticated ways to communicate are not the only human particularities, we must consider to explain how our ancestors have colonised the whole planet. Factors that promote cooperative and satisfying relationships are also undoubtedly essential. This is why we must give importance to studies of the recent evolution of the capacity for empathy. At the annual meeting of the Association for Psychological Science, in June 2010, a synthesis of 72 studies of the evolution of personality traits of American students (college graduates) between 1979 and 2009 was presented.[19] According to this research, college graduates are 40% less empathetic than those of three or four decades ago. The decline has been progressive, particularly after the year 2000. These studies have a great scientific value because they used data from people who were from the same age group but different birth cohorts. I already had the opportunity to emphasise that, until now, the advent of modern obstetrics has not been considered to interpret several kinds of recent and spectacular transformations of our species.[20]

In Which Court Is the Ball?

The ball is undoubtedly in the court of epidemiologists. Until now, the possible long-term effects of new interferences in the period of birth preparation could not have been considered: it will undoubtedly take a long time before explorations of risk factors for pathological conditions in old age are feasible, since the most significant turning point in the history of obstetrics took place at the end of the second half of the 20th century. I am thinking, in particular, of neurodegenerative and cardiovascular diseases. I am also thinking of life expectancy.

However, many studies about possible middle-term issues we have already mentioned are theoretically possible without waiting too long and without overcoming unprecedented methodological challenges. This is the case of sexual orientation, intellectual quotient or capacity for empathy. We can even imagine that some preliminary enquiries might immediately provide valuable indications about plausible cause and effect relationships between what happens in the period surrounding birth — including "birth preparation" — and pathological conditions or personality traits later on in life. Let us imagine, for example, that labour induction and pre-labour caesarean sections appear as risk factors for the same pathological conditions. The physiological states associated with these two obstetrical interventions are different. Pre-labour caesarean sections are associated with a state of stress deprivation, while labour induction is usually associated with prolonged pharmacological assistance. If these two ways to interrupt the phase of birth preparation appear as risk factors for the same diseases, it will be worth going deeper into a probable cause and effect relationship.

Anyway, the task of epidemiologists will be arduous. They will need to associate sophisticated appropriate statistical strategies for dealing with "multiplicity" and for reducing the likelihood that a chance association could be deemed causal. After raising questions about the development of futurology, as an emerging scientific discipline, we'll imagine the time when a reliable "biological clock", such as the "epigenetic clock", will make it easy to compare chronological age and physiological age. This is a promising way to complete conventional epidemiology and to study, in particular, life expectancy in relation to what happened during the primal period.

Meanwhile, one can imagine several scenarios. One of them would start with the sudden emergence of a new awareness leading to encourage cautious strategies before we know more. Another one would be to passively wait for hard data before reconsidering the dominant medical attitudes. If the second scenario prevails, there is a future for the sorcerer's apprentice.

References

1. Kawai K, Gebremeskel BG and Acosta CJ (2014) Systematic review of incidence and complications of herpes zoster: towards a global perspective. *BMJ Open* **4(6)**:e004833. doi.org/10.1136/bmjopen-2014-004833.
2. Hales CM, Harpaz R, Joesoef MR and Bialek SR (2013) Examination of links between herpes zoster incidence and childhood varicella vaccination. *Ann Intern Med* **159**:739–45.
3. Leung J, Harpaz R, Molinari NA, *et al.* (2011) Herpes zoster incidence among insured persons in the United States, 1993–2006: Evaluation of impact of varicella vaccination. *Clin Infect Dis* **52**:332–40.
4. Brisson M, Edmunds WJ, Law B *et al.* (2001) Epidemiology of varicella zoster virus infection in Canada and the United Kingdom. *Epidemiol Infect* **127**:305–14.
5. Pérez-Farinós N, Ordobás M, García-Fernández C, *et al.* (2004) Varicella and herpes zoster in Madrid, based on the Sentinel General Practitioner Network: 1997–2004. *BMC Infect Dis* **7**:59.
6. Toyama N, Shiraki K and Society of the Miyazaki Prefecture Dermatologists (2009) Epidemiology of herpes zoster and its relationship to varicella in Japan: a 10-year survey of 48,388 herpes zoster cases in Miyazaki prefecture. *J Med Virol* **81**:2053–8.
7. Chao DY, Chien YZ, Yeh YP, *et al.* (2012) The incidence of varicella and herpes zoster in Taiwan during a period of increasing varicella vaccine coverage, 2000–2008. *Epidemiol Infect* **140**:1131–40.
8. Wu PY, Wu HD, Chou TC and Sung FC (2013) Varicella vaccination alters the chronological trends of herpes zoster and varicella. *PLoS One* **8**:e77709.
9. Jardine A, Conaty SJ and Vally H (2011) Herpes zoster in Australia: evidence of increase in incidence in adults attributable to varicella immunization? *Epidemiol Infect* **139**:658–65.

10. Russell ML, Schopflocher DP, Svenson L and Virani SN (2007) Secular trends in the epidemiology of shingles in Alberta. *Epidemiol Infect* **135**:908–13.

11. Esteban-Vasallo MD, Gil-Prieto R, Domínguez-Berjón MF, *et al.* (2014) Temporal trends in incidence rates of herpes zoster among patients treated in primary care centers in Madrid (Spain), 2005–2012. *J Infect* **68**:378–86.

12. Rimland D and Moanna A (2010) Increasing incidence of herpes zoster among veterans. *Clin Infect Dis* **50**:1000–5.

13. Kawai K, Yawn BP, Wollan P and Harpaz R (2016) Increasing Incidence of Herpes Zoster Over a 60-year Period From a Population-based Study. *Clin Infect Dis* **63(2)**:221–6. doi: 10.1093/cid/ciw296.

14. Marin M, Harpaz R, Zhang J, *et al.* (2016) Risk Factors for Herpes Zoster Among Adults. *Open Forum Infect Dis* **3(3)**:ofw119. doi: 10.1093/ofid/ofw119. eCollection 2016 Sep.

15. Flynn JR (1987) Massive IQ gains in 14 nations. *Psychol Bull* **101**: 171–91.

16. Trahan LH, Stuebing KK, Fletcher JM and Hiscock M (2014) The Flynn effect: a meta-analysis. *Psychol Bull* **140(5)**:1332–60. doi: 10.1037/a0037173.

17. Bratsberg B and Rogeberg O (2018) Flynn effect and its reversal are both environmentally caused. *PNAS* **115(26)**:6674–78. doi: 10.1073/pnas.1718793115.

18. Horizon documentary (1975) A Time to be Born. *BBC*. Available at: www.bbc.co.uk/iplayer/episode/p01z4pcy/horizon-19741975-a-time-to-be-born.

19. Konrath SH, O'Brien EH and Hsing C (2011) Changes in dispositional empathy in American college students over time: a meta-analysis. *Pers Soc Psychol Review* **15(2)**:180–98. doi: 10.1177/1088868310377395.

20. Odent M (2014) The future of the human oxytocin system. In: *Childbirth and the Evolution of Homo sapiens*. Pinter & Martin, London.

12 The Future of Lullabies

Abstract

Modes of communication in the period surrounding birth have been described but not scientifically investigated. This is the case of "motherese" ("baby talk"). Its universal characteristics lead us to conclude that it is associated with a reduced cultural conditioning and therefore a reduced neocortical control. This is also the case of lullabies, as universal variants of baby talk: an authentic lullaby is improvised at a time when the mother is still in a specific physiological state. Studies of the roots of the words reveal that in many languages the word that means "lullaby" is conveying the intention to calm down, while in other languages the focus is on the rocking movements. We enlarge the topic by presenting improvised and therefore authentic lullabies as prototypical forms of spontaneous creative behaviour. This is an opportunity to mention that, according to studies through brain imaging, musical improvisation is characterised by a reduced neocortical activity.

This is an obligatory topic for students in human nature who understand Homo as a primate endowed of the capacity to develop sophisticated ways to communicate.

As we previously mentioned, the way human births are physiologically prepared could not be understood as long as the concept of neocortical inhibition was not assimilated. We must open a parenthesis to emphasise that, after the birth, the maternal neocortex does not come back overnight to its baseline activity. This is confirmed by the particularities of post-partum modes of communication: they have been described but not scientifically investigated.

Baby Talk

During the days following birth, mothers — particularly those who have not used pharmacological assistance and don't feel observed — have a well-known tendency to spontaneously communicate with their baby through "baby talk", often called "motherese". "Motherese" has a special pattern of intonation. The mother is talking in a high-pitched voice. The words are fully articulated. The speech is slowed with a great number of pauses. The sentences are short and often repeated. There is a wide opening of the mouth. There are usually body movements, particularly head movements that stress certain syllables. Since this simplified language has universal characteristics, one can conclude that it is associated with a reduced cultural conditioning. In other words, this mode of communication is not restrained by a powerful neocortical control.

From Lullabies to "Berceuses"

Lullabies may be presented as universal variants of baby talk. An authentic lullaby is not composed by a third party. It is improvised at a time when the mother is still in a specific physiological state. It is not accompanied by instruments. The music is simple and repetitive, with long sections between pauses.

After thousands of years of socialisation of childbirth, invasive beliefs and rituals have interfered in the mother–baby interaction at such a point that historical studies have a limited interest. Their vocation is to look at variants of the domination of nature since the

"Neolithic revolution". As a general rule, newborn babies have not been in the arms of their mother. They were not in a position to identify the voice of their mother. Immediate tight swaddling was a widespread way to neutralise the archaic sense of touching.

However, we can learn from other perspectives, particularly studies of the roots of the words. Interestingly, the word commonly used in English (lullaby) has not the same etymological roots, and therefore the same original meaning as the words commonly used in many other languages. The English word, and also the Russian "bayukat", the Serbo-Croatian "uspavanka" and the Arabic "tah-wida" are conveying an intention (to lull, to soothe, to calm down). The Spanish word "cancion de cuna", the German "wiegenfield" are descriptive of the context (cradle song).

Today, while there is a renewed scientific interest in the develop-ment of human sensory functions, it is notable that in a great diversity of languages the focus is on the rocking movements. This is the case of the Russian word "kolybel'naia", the Czech "ukolébavka", the Armenian "ororots" and the French "berceuse". "Berceuse" prob-ably comes from barbaric Latin "berciolus", derived from "berto", a verb suggestive of the action of moving by turning.[1]

The history of furniture confirms that it has been understood for ages that babies need to be rocked. There is evidence that in France, in the Carolingian era, babies could easily be rocked in especially designed cradles made of tree-trunks.[2] After referring to these perspectives suggesting the importance given to the rocking movements, we'll add that the tempos of lullabies tend to be slow, and that, rhythmically, there are shared patterns. Lullabies are usually in triple or 6/8 time, inducing a characteristic swinging or rocking motion. It has been underlined that this is a way to mimic what the baby can perceive in the womb as the mother moves.

The deep-rooted importance given to rocking movements is noteworthy at a time when it is still commonplace to refer to the well-established list of "the five senses": touching, hearing, smelling, tasting and seeing. The expression "sixth sense" suggests that there is only one additional sense besides the traditional list: it refers to extrasensory perception of information not gained through the five recognised senses. There is a mysterious cultural tendency to ignore the most primitive and the most universal sensory functions, which are the basis of the sense of balance, of spatial orientation and adaptation to gravity. It is still commonplace to forget at which point we are dependent on the functions of the inner ear (the vestibular system). In 1981, I participated in a collective book in French about the development of human sensory functions. During a preliminary editorial meeting we had established a list of authoritative experts who could write about "the five senses". At the end of the meeting, when we were ready to go, I just asked a question: "Et le système vestibulaire?" (what about the vestibular system?). This is how, in spite of my low degree of competence, I was asked to write a paper on this topic.[3]

Our comments about lullabies are opportunities to emphasise once more the importance of interdisciplinary perspectives to study universal aspects of human nature. In the age of overspecialisation, it is unusual, for example, to combine what we can learn from etymology (the roots of the words), what we can learn from the history of furniture and what we can learn from physiology. We'll complete this overview by recalling that the ear is the only organ of the human body that can reach nearly its adult size during foetal life. By associating appropriate kinds of sounds and rocking movements, lullabies stimulate both the external ear (sense of hearing) and the inner ear (adaptation to gravity and sense of balance). In other words, authentic lullabies satisfy basic human needs at an important phase of development.

As students of human nature, we'll even dare to present improvised and therefore authentic lullabies as prototypical forms of spontaneous creative behaviour. There have already been attempts to study artistic creativity from physiological perspectives. By using

Magnetic Resonance Imaging, the authors of a valuable study investigated improvisation in jazz pianists. They found that improvisation (compared with production of learned musical sequences) was consistently characterised by a "transient hypofrontality".[4] This means, in practice, an extensive deactivation of the prefrontal cortex. It is not different to what we call, to simplify, a reduced neocortical control. It is worth underlining that when a mother is improvising a lullaby after releasing an appropriate powerful hormonal flow, she is an obvious state of "transient hypofrontality". There are significant anecdotes of women who, after giving birth without cultural assistance, could not remember having unexpectedly sung improvised lullabies. One can wonder for how long after birth, a state of hypofrontality might remain detectable. According to a magnetic resonance imaging study of parents watching videos of their own 4- to 6-months old baby playing, mothers (but not fathers) showed an activation of amygdala (a primitive part of the brain).[5]

Joy

One of the effects — and probably functions — of authentic lullabies is also to transmit emotional states.

I am tempted to suggest that the most common messages expressed that way belong to the family of transcendent emotional states. Once a mother told me that she saw the whole universe in the eyes of her newborn baby. My own mother used to say that the day of my birth had been the most joyful day of her life. I have therefore personal reasons to include "joy" in this family of emotions. There is a major obstacle in studying "joy" from a scientific perspective. It is that until now keywords such as "anxiety, "stress", "depression", "psychological distress" or fear" are much more productive than the keyword "joy".

This is why we must refer to what we can learn from artists, who often precede scientists. It is significant that, in general, artists associate "joy" with emergence of life and transcendence. In one of her poems, my mother wrote: "Un grand hymne à la joie évoque le Tres-Haut", which can be translated as "A grand hymn of joy evokes the Almighty".[6] The poem includes the words "printemps" (spring), "oiseau qui chante" (singing bird), "enfant" (child). "The Ode to Joy" — now the European anthem — is also highly significant. It is based on the fourth movement of Beethoven's 9th symphony. One can wonder how the music evokes joy…sudden intermittent series of ascending notes are undoubtedly suggestive of the emergence of life. The original text of the European anthem was the poem written by Friedrich Schiller at the end of the 18th century. From the start of the poem, joy is presented as sudden access to the divine: "Freude, schöner Götterfunken" (Joy, beautiful spark of divinity).

The Future

Is there a future for lullabies, for artistic creativity…for joy?

References

1. *Dictionnaire National* (1852). Simon et Garnier, editeurs, Paris.
2. Eugene Viollet-le-Duc. Dictionnaire raisonné du mobilier français de l'époque carolingienne a la Renaissance. *Librairie centrale d'architecture 1873–1874* 1:37–9.
3. Michel Odent (1981) Et le système vestibulaire? In: *Les cahiers du nouveau-né*. Stock, Paris.
4. Limb CJ and Braun AR (2008) Neural substrates of spontaneous musical performance: an FMRI study of jazz improvisation. *PLoS One* **3(2)**:e1679. doi: 10.1371/journal.pone.0001679.
5. Atzil S, Hendler T, Zagoory-Sharon O, *et al.* (2012) Synchrony and specificity in the maternal and the paternal brain: relations to oxytocin and vasopressin. *J Am Acad Child Adolesc* **51(8)**:798–811. doi: 10.1016/j.jaac.2012.06.008.
6. Madeleine Odent (1978) Joie. In: *Rayons du soir*. Les Presses du Monteil, Pessac.

13 The Future of Transcendent Emotional States

Abstract

After having introduced the concept of the "Scientification of Love", I introduce the concept of the "Scientification of Transcendence". Studies of emotional states that give access to another reality than space and time reality cannot be dissociated from studies of subjective experiences originally associated with episodes of human reproductive life: "foetus ejection reflex", "milk ejection reflex", and "sperm ejection reflex".

Not only from physiological perspectives, but also from historical perspectives, human reproduction and transcendent emotional states are indissociable topics. They can be looked at in the framework of the domination of nature that started about ten millennia ago and that includes the domestication of plants and animals, and also a certain degree of domestication of Homo.

This chapter provides an opportunity to shed new light on the functions of emotions.

Our comments on lullabies and other modes of communication in the period surrounding birth have inspired questions about transcendent emotional states. I'll go one step further and introduce the concept of "Scientification of Transcendence" after having introduced, in the past, the concept of "Scientification of Love".[1]

Emotional states providing access to another reality than space and time reality seem to be inherent in human nature. At the present time, the keyword "transcendence" leads to the work of philosophers, anthropologists interested in beliefs and rituals, and theologians. It does not appear in the framework of emotional states. This is not special to our current cultural milieu. In Aristotle's rhetoric (4th century BC), it was not mentioned among the eight basic human emotions. More recently, in "The Expression of Emotions in Man and Animals" (1872), Charles Darwin has not modified the limits of the topic.

The Scientification of Transcendence

In a renewed scientific context, it suddenly appears inevitable to integrate access to transcendence into the framework of human emotional states. Transcendent emotional states are less mysterious at a time when everybody has heard about the properties of messengers such as endorphins and oxytocin, while sophisticated techniques of brain imaging are developing.

The prerequisite for the "scientification of transcendence" is the development of new ways of thinking with the help of a simplified vocabulary. By focusing on a small number of terms such as "transcendence", "emotional states" and "scientification" we avoid difficult to define terms that transmit the dominant cultural conditioning. This is the case of "spirituality", which implies the concept of "spirit" as the animating and vital principle in man and animals. This is the case of "religiosity", which has been evaluated through variables such as church attendance. This is the case of "mysticism", which is often linked with one particular established religion. This is also the case of "self-transcendence", which is the capacity to expand self-boundaries rather than to have access to an out of space and time reality. Nearly a century ago, Carl Jung already expressed warnings about the overuse of difficult to define terms. In a lecture delivered to the literary Society of Augsburg, he said about "spirit": "Are we sure that when we use this word we all mean the same thing?"

We are now in a position to offer preliminary interpretations. We have at our disposal recently acquired knowledge regarding ecstatic states in general. This is leading us to mention subjective experiences originally associated with episodes of human reproductive life: "foetus ejection reflex", "milk ejection reflex", "sperm ejection reflex", etc.[2]

The point is to accept that human reproduction and transcendent emotional states are indissociable topics one can explore through emerging and fast developing scientific disciplines.

The Limits of the Domination of Nature

The links between these topics are obvious, not only in the light of modern physiology, but also from an historical perspective. The organisation, the regulation, and the socialisation of human physiological functions related to reproduction are historically associated with the control of the paths to transcendence. While mating was organised and ritualised, and while childbirth was socialised, access to transcendence was organised. All societies develop, promote, and give direction to a limited number of easy to control paths towards transcendence that are culturally acceptable. This is how we can understand, for example, the functions of prayer, religious music, fasting, psychedelic drugs and hypnotic trances. One of the effects of the cultural control of genital sexuality, childbirth, lactation and access to transcendence has been the association of orgasmic states with the concepts of shame, culpability and fear.

These considerations about transcendent emotional states offer perfect opportunities to focus on the need for unifying visions of traditionally and artificially separated topics. Studying lullabies led us to mention the expression of emotions, including transcendent emotional states. Then we found it impossible to consider such emotional states without referring to the subjective experiences associated with phases of human reproductive life. This led us to recall that the domination of nature that started about ten millennia ago included not only the domestication of plants and animals, but also a certain degree of domestication of Homo. Finally, we were obliged to realise that we have reached the limits of the domination of nature. More than ever we need to explore the future. What is the future of transcendent emotional states?

The Future of the Sense of Humour

We might raise similar questions about all human emotional states. Once more we need unifying visions of traditionally separated topics. We are in a position to understand that specific fluctuations of neocortical control are part and parcel of emotional states. This has not been understood until now. In the case of anger, for example, an emotional state that has been comparatively well studied for a long time, the focus has always been on the activation of the hypothalamic–pituitary–adrenal axis and catecholamine release. If, in the future, the focus is on fluctuations of neocortical control, there will be new reasons and new ways to study anger. There will be reasons, for example, to study in depth tantrums, as frequent variants of anger at an age when the neocortex has not reached its final phase of development. What are the functions of tantrums? New ways of thinking inspire unusual questions.

During the 16th century, François Rabelais, an interdisciplinary student of human nature, gave great importance to laughing and the sense of humour, two related topics. As a medical doctor, long before the age of evidence-based medicine, he developed "gelototherapy", relying on the healing effects of laughing.[3] Thanks to him, it is usually accepted that to laugh is proper to man ("le rire est le propre de l'homme"). Today we must take into account that it is associated with obvious fluctuations of neocortical control. The

French term "fou rire" is an eloquent way to emphasise how uncontrollable a fit of laughter can be. At a time when neocortical inhibition appears as a key to understanding human nature, this implies that any exploration of the future of Homo must include questions about the evolution of the capacity to laugh in the framework of the ability to occasionally escape from daily reality through emotions.

It is now understood that, in adverse situations, the best way to protect one's health is to escape, if fight is impossible. In-depth studies of emotions, as ways to escape, will become essential to suggest preliminary answers to questions about the future of human health.

I am already collecting data about laughing induction in the framework of "The scientification of the sense of humour". One of the oldest studies in this framework was published as early as 2013 by authoritative researchers from the prestigious Stanford University.[4]

Meanwhile we understand those who prefer to avoid the term "scientification" and maintain "love", "transcendence" and "sense of humour" in the framework of mysteries. Is the need for mysteries a universal human trait?

References

1. Odent M (1999) *The Scientification of Love*. Free Association Books, London.
2. Odent M (2009) *The Functions of the Orgasms: the highways to Transcendence*. Pinter & Martin, London.
3. Odent M (1999) In Lifeline. *Lancet* **353**:764. doi.org/10.1016/S0140-6736(05)76145-6.
4. Vrticka P, Black JM and Reiss AL (2013) The neural basis of humour processing. *Natl Rev Neurosci* **14(12)**:860–8. doi: 10.1038/nrn3566.

Chapter **14** From Language Absorption to Language Learning

Abstract

After contrasting language absorption and language learning, we are in a position to rephrase questions about the development of analytic thinking versus "synthesising thinking". These are essential questions in the age of overspecialisation and fast evolution of spoken and written languages.

The Case of Written Language

The career of my mother — as a teacher in the French state school system — started at the beginning of World War I. When I was born, in 1930, she was in charge of "une école maternelle" (a school for children aged two to six). This is why I acquired the capacity to read in a way that was radically challenging the standardised attitudes. My mother had understood from experience that very young, human beings have developed their brain and their sense of sight in such a way that they are able to easily remember a whole written word as a picture with a meaning. We can say in retrospect that, as early as in the early 1930s, I had acquired the ability to read and write through a "global method". It is as if I could photograph words.

After the age of six, I went to the primary school of the village. At that age, I was mature enough to learn to read by breaking the words into their formal elements, which are letters and syllabi. I became gradually mature enough to use punctuation, as a substitute for intonation, rhythm and gestures that are essential components of spoken language: an association of written words can transmit different messages if it is followed by a simple interruption (full stop, comma, semicolon) or by an ellipsis, an exclamation mark, or a question mark. After the age of 12, in a secondary school, I studied ancient languages (Latin and Greek) and English. I developed a keen interest in Latin. I was probably developing my analytic mind mostly through comparative studies of Latin versus French grammar and syntax.

Long after, I had conversations with my mother about how written word can be "absorbed" before being learned. It is an inescapable topic for students of human nature. It is probable that the syllabic method plays an important role in the development of analytic thinking, which could be defined as the capacity to divide the whole into different parts. But human creativity relies on all other ways of thinking. The opposite of analytic thinking is, literally, "synthesising thinking". This concept is vague. We may present it as an umbrella term. It includes intuition. It includes "lateral thinking", as the capacity to look at a situation or problem from an unexpected point of view. It includes opinion-based critical thinking. At a time when the negative side effects of overspecialisation are perceived, and when we are constantly facing new situations, it seems urgent to try to tip the balance between different ways of thinking. Should we favour the phase of written language absorption? Once more, in unprecedented situations, we must first phrase new questions.

Our comments are expressed in Europe, where most languages belong to the Indo-European family. It is notable that, even between narrowly related European languages, there are significant differences where written words are concerned. Written languages are more or less phonetic. Written French is less phonetic than Spanish. This implies that, when we speak French, many phonetically similar words cannot be understood if extracted from a context. For example, the word that means "faith" (foi), the word that means "liver" (foie), a word that refers to a French city (Foix) and a word that means "time" (once = une fois) are phonetically similar. Since the "Great vowel shift" of the 15th and 16th century, English spellings often deviate from their representation in pronunciation. One can conclude that written language acquisition is a complex issue that cannot follow universal rules.

We must also keep in mind that in some parts of the world the structures of written languages are radically different. For example, written Chinese is not based on an alphabet or a compact syllabary. Instead, the components of Chinese characters may depict objects or represent abstract notions. The issues are also special in languages without vowels. This is the case of languages derived from Aramaic (Hebrew, Arabic and Syrian). Even if, according to influential modern linguistic theories based on the genetic component of the language faculty, there is a "universal grammar", we must acknowledge radical variations where the written expression is concerned.

Prenatal Language Absorption

There are several reasons why I first introduced the case of written language, rather than spoken language. The first reason is that the capacity to read and write is an aspect of our modern lifestyle, since it became recently widespread all over the world. The second reason is that studying written language acquisition is an easy way to contrast absorption and learning. Furthermore, in the age of overspecialisation, we must jump on opportunities to raise questions about the development of the "synthesising way of thinking".

About spoken language, I'll just introduce a chapter of this enormous topic. Once more, our objective is to illustrate the concept of absorption. There is an accumulation of recent data about exposure to language during foetal life. It is well accepted today that human beings start absorbing their mother tongue before being born, as soon as the peripheral auditory system is fully formed. Newborn babies show a preference for their mother's voice at birth and babies of monolingual mothers prefer to listen to their native language over an unfamiliar language.[1] In other words, it appears that human beings learn about the properties of the native language while still in the womb. These facts have inspired studies with near infrared spectroscopy to clarify how prenatal experience might shape the brain response to language.[2] It appeared that language familiarity has a bilateral effect on the brain responses.

For many reasons, we are expecting a fast evolution of spoken and written languages. The first reason is that, in the age of cheap modes of locomotion, intercultural breeding is more and more common: many children develop in families where several languages are used. In such families, the frontiers between absorbed language and learned language cannot be precise. A related reason is that after absorbing their mother tongue, hundreds of thousands of 21st century human beings, all over the world, are learning English as the lingua franca. It is furthermore obvious that computers and smartphones are transforming in a spectacular way both oral and written modes of expression.

Acquisition of language should become a central topic for futurologists.

References

1. DeCasper AJ and Fifer WP (1980) Of human bonding: newborns prefer their mothers' voices. *Science* **208(4448)**:1174–6.
2. May L, Byers-Heinlein K, Gervain J and Werker JF (2011) Language and the newborn brain: does prenatal language experience shape the neonate neural response to speech? *Front Psychol* **2**:222. doi: 10.3389/fpsyg.2011.00222.

Chapter 15

The Future of Futurology

Abstract

When studying the perinatal period as a critical phase of individual development, we are constantly turned towards the future. We cannot ignore futurology as an emerging scientific discipline. After considering established knowledge regarding the past and the present, futurologists explore the future. Their keywords are extrapolation, projection, probability, anticipation and plausibility. There are already future-oriented scientific disciplines such as demography, climatology and geology (with new concepts such as "Great acceleration" and "Anthropocene"). In spite of precise and easily summarised definitions, the frontier between futurology and science fiction remains blurred and needs to be clarified. It is notable that, until now, futurologists have considered the effects of human actions without raising useful questions about probable transformations of Homo. One cannot pronounce on the future of futurology without analysing this paradox.

The function of this new discipline is to explore the future. Its keywords are extrapolation, projection, anticipation, probability and plausibility. After considering established knowledge regarding the past and the present, futurologists study the future. This scientific discipline started immediately after World War II. This is the time when the term "futurology" was coined in Germany by Ossip Flechtheim.[1]

Futurology, based on a new way of thinking, has immediately influenced several kinds of specialised experts in emerging disciplines. This is the case of demographists, who study the growth and density of populations and offer anticipations based mostly on projections and extrapolations. This is the case of modern meteorologists and climatologists. This is also the case of geologists, who designate the "Anthropocene" as the new geological epoch characterised by unprecedented alterations of the planet by human activities. Futurology is becoming vital, at a time when, for obvious reasons, human beings must train themselves to develop their prospective thinking.

From Imagination to Exploration

In spite of precise and easily summarised definitions, the frontier between futurology and science fiction often remains blurred. Let us recall that science fiction is supposed to belong to the framework of arts, particularly literature. It is precisely because the frontier is blurred that it needs to be clarified. The imagination of writers and other artists interested in the future has always been fed by available contemporary scientific knowledge. On the other hand, scientists, as human beings, are also endowed with imagination. They need imagination to elaborate and propose for further investigations and testable hypotheses.

From a historical perspective, it is notable that the advent of futurology, at the end of World War II, coincided with the disappearance of active groups of science fiction fans, such as the "Futurians".

Interestingly, science fiction remains powerful and influential whatever the scientific context: it is so ancient that it belongs to the bases of our cultural conditioning, like myths and legends. It probably started with poems that were more likely intended to be heard than read.

Let us recall, for example, that "A True Story" was written in the second century AD by Lucian of Samosata, a Greek speaking author of Syrian descent. It includes themes such as travel to other worlds, extraterrestrial lifeforms, interplanetary warfare, and artificial life. It is significant that Jules Verne, as a French novelist in the 19th century, has been one of the most translated authors in the world, ranking between Agatha Christie and William Shakespeare. Jules Verne was the author of books with significant titles, such as "Journey to the Centre of the Earth", "Twenty Thousand Leagues under the Sea" and "Around the World in Eighty Days". The links between science fiction and scientific activity appear strong from an historical perspective. There has been a scientific golden age for the Middle East: we have mentioned the name of Lucian of Samosata in such a context. There has been a golden age for Western Europe: we have mentioned Jules Vernes. There has been a golden age for North America, during the twentieth century. Today intense scientific productivity has a tendency to move towards Asia: it is notable that the acclaimed novel and the acclaimed film "The Wandering Earth" are Chinese.

The issue of communication with extraterrestrials is typical of the current period of transition. At the turn of the century, "Triad", the novel published by Sheila Finch, who had coined the term "xenolinguistics", was unanimously classified as pure fiction.[2] Today Sheri Wells-Jensen, an academic linguist from Bowling Green State University, may attract the attention of a prestigious scientific journal such as Nature about her workshops on alien linguistics, while Scientific American may introduce the issue of Alien interpreters.[3,4] It would have been considered a joke, until recently, to mention that New Scientist has published a paper about "how to decipher alien tongues" and that the NASA Astrobiology Institute, University of Washington, has written about "Earth linguistics, xenolinguistics, and the possibility of communication".[5,6] To illustrate the amplitude of the phenomenon, we'll mention that the current network of alien hunters comprises the "Search for Extraterrestrial Intelligence" (SETI). SETI, a key research contractor to NASA and the National Science Foundation, employs more than 130 scientists, educators, and administrative staff. Fad or authentic futurology?

Futurology Today

Many themes that have been specific to the realm of fiction since time immemorial have suddenly extended across the frontier and are invading the growing realm of authentic futurology. Today, when reading about the world's first floating city that is set to appear in the Pacific Ocean off the island of Tahiti in the 2020s, one cannot help thinking of how, according to Homer, Odysseus and a team of "Homo navigators" found an island floating above the sea: it was the island of Aeolia, home of Aeolus, god of wind.

We may also mention the studies of planet-to-space transportation systems. We have entered a new historical phase since the "International Space Elevator Consortium" (ISEC) was formed in 2008. The objective is to promote the development, construction, and operation of a space elevator as a "revolutionary and efficient way to space for all humanity".

The most breathtaking project — dubbed Breakthrough Starshot — was announced in April 2016. The masterminds behind the plan are the celebrity physicist Stephen Hawking (who died in 2018), the Facebook founder Mark Zuckerberg, and the Russian billionaire Yuri Milner. The objective is to launch a swarm of probes the size of postage stamps into outer space at 20% the speed of light. The destination is our nearest galactic neighbours, a star system called Alpha Centauri. It would be a flyby mission to reach Alpha Centauri in just over 20 years from launch, beaming home images of its recently discovered planet Proxima b, and any other planet that may lie in the system, as well as collecting other scientific data such as analysis of magnetic fields. A preliminary $100 million research and engineering programme will seek proof of concept. Of course, for naïve lay persons, it may seem more realistic, in the foreseeable future, to focus on plans to establish bases on the Moon and Mars. Perhaps the project of sending human beings out of the solar system should remain in the framework of dreams. It is outside the field of futurology. Futurologists are classified as serious and respectable scientists.

The study of techniques facilitating communication between Earth people is another important branch of authentic futurology: universal translators, telepathy, telekinesis and holographic TVs are on the list of emerging topics. On the same list, one can include techniques facilitating transportation in daily life: driverless cars and flying cars, thanks to magnetic levitation, for example. The replacement of fossil sources of energy and carbon removal technologies are inescapable fields of futurology. While we are experiencing the most rapid technological revolution in history, there is a future for futurologists.

Futurology and Obstetrics

We would need volumes to present an overview of countless articles and books anticipating plausible spectacular advances in curative medicine. This is why we'll remain within the limited framework of obstetrics, the point of departure of our exploration of the future of Homo. Since obstetrical practices are related to the health of very young human beings with a life expectancy of about 80 years, it is the medical specialty futurologists should be focusing on. One of the bases of obstetrics today is substitutive pharmacological assistance. This simply means that when labouring women cannot efficiently release their natural hormones they rely on pharmacological substitutes. In practice it means that a great proportion of women give birth with drips of synthetic oxytocin replacing the natural hormone and synthetic morphine-like substances replacing the so-called endorphins.

Until now, the highly plausible long-term negative side effects of synthetic oxytocin during the birth process have not been evaluated by epidemiologists. We can make similar comments about drugs of the morphine family, particularly fentanyl — usually administered in the epidural space. It has been demonstrated that a certain amount of fentanyl is reaching the baby during an epidural analgesia. There have even been evaluations of the transfer of fentanyl from the maternal epidural space to the foetal blood stream. Concentrations of 0.077 ng/mL have been found in the blood of the umbilical vein after epidural analgesia.[7] Although fentanyl is 800 times more lipo-soluble than morphine, we must keep in mind that it is 100 times more potent. While short-term effects of exposure to fentanyl cannot easily be detected immediately after birth, we must remain cautious while waiting for long-term epidemiological studies considering a great diversity of issues such as drug addiction, suicidal behaviour, sexual orientation, and prevalence of non-communicable diseases in adulthood.

Let us imagine that, through a new generation of epidemi-ological studies, it appears that current methods of substitutive pharmacology have unacceptable long-term negative side effects. Let us imagine, at the same time, that the concept of neocortical inhibition has been assimilated and popularised and that birth physiology is first and foremost understood as a chapter of brain physiology. There would suddenly be reasons to explore radically new kinds of medical assistance in childbirth. The bases of renewed strategies might lead to rely on states of transient "hypofrontality". In other words, the objective would be to reduce neocortical control. Instead of replacing the hormones involved in the birth process, the objective would be to facilitate their release. In fact, such strat-egies would not be absolutely new. In many cultures and from time immemorial, shamans have used psychedelic drugs when involved in difficult births. We must also learn from labouring women who are in occasional or pathological states of "hypofrontality": women in a vegetative coma, for example, don't need pharmacological assistance to give birth.

My personal understanding of the effects of typical states of "hypofrontality" has been occasionally reactivated through anecdotes. Once a woman had a spectacular foetus ejection reflex after drinking a whole glass of champagne. Champagne is a very special wine: thanks to the bubbles, the alcohol it contains is immediately brought to the brain. I also learnt from the easy way schizophrenic women with neocortical inhibition deficits used to give birth before the widespread adoption of powerful antipsychotic treatments. I cannot forget that I started to understand birth physiology in the early 1960s, when a friend of mine, working for a pharmaceutical firm, asked me to test during labour the effect of the inhibitory neuromediator gamma-hydroxybutyric acid (GHB): he had been told that GHB had oxytocic effects. I understood that it did not work like oxytocin, but facilitated its release by reducing neocortical activity.

It is still premature to pronounce on the acceptable ways — pharmacological or physical — to induce transitory states of reduced neocortical control. The point is to realise that obstetrics, more than curative medicine, should become a central topic for futurologists.

Futurology Tomorrow

The emerging disciplines that we include in the framework of futurology must overcome difficulties that could not be easily identified in the past. We'll just consider the case of demography, as a typical example. Although demographic thoughts are traced back to antiquity, particularly Greece, Rome, China and India, we arbitrarily consider that demography, as a branch of futurology, started after World War II: a key event had been the launching of the "International Union for the Scientific Study of Populations" at an assembly held in Washington in 1947.

Until now, anticipations established by demographists have been based on simple projections and extrapolations from easily available data. For example, according to UN projections, the world population will reach about 9 billion in 2075. There are reasons to be sceptical about these projections. We are reaching a turning point when unexpected facts lead us to reconsider the comparative importance of factors that should be taken into account in demographic anticipations.

As an example of such facts, we'll mention that the total number of births in mainland China in 2018 was around 15 million: it was still 17.2 million in 2017. This spectacular decline is surprising if we consider that laws starting in January 2016 put an end to the one child per couple policy. It is notable that similar demographic tendencies were reported in Hong Kong and Taiwan, where there has never been the equivalent of the one child per couple legislation. It is obvious that political decision makers have a limited power in terms of demographic fluctuations. We might make similar comments about the comparative importance usually given to several factors that have already been included in demographic projections in countries that share modern lifestyles. This is the case of female labour participation, urban versus rural residence, birth control usage, female and male age, and religiosity.

Without detailed analyses and tentative interpretations of recent unexpected facts, we can simply observe that the anticipations provided by demographists do not consider the way babies are born, although it is the aspect of lifestyle that has been the most dramatically modified within some decades, and although the period surrounding birth appears critical in the formation of individuals. We'll just emphasise that mainland China, Hong Kong and Taiwan share the same skyrocketing rates of caesarean sections and the same demographic tendencies. We might enlarge the topic and mention, for example, that compared with other European countries, Italy is characterised by both the lowest fertility rates and very high rates of caesarean sections.

We don't need long developments to convince anyone that there are reasons to introduce obstetrical practices among the factors that may influence demographic fluctuations. The prerequisite for such a new step is to realise that most women don't actively give birth in the age of safe caesarean sections and pharmacological substitutes for natural hormones. This fact should inspire questions about human reproductivity in the future, in relation to the modes of birth. In a radically new context, a prominent place must be given, inside the concept of reproductivity, to the desire or the urge to survive through procreation. This is an example of an unavoidable new question that should prevail upon many others: what is the degree of reproductivity of a population born by caesarean section?

In the age of overspecialisation, the links are not yet perceived between demography and sexology. How to combine two ways of thinking? On the one hand, demographists are constantly working with numbers. The field of sexuality, on the other hand, is outside the field of rationality: the urge to transmit one's genes is not rational. How to associate demography and sexology in the framework of futurology?

There are many ways to try to explain why, until now, futurologists have explored the effects of human actions without considering possible transformations of Homo.

What kind of human beings will inhabit planet Earth in the future?

We cannot pronounce on the future of futurology without starting from this question.

References

1. Flechtheim OK (1945) Teaching the Future. *Journal of Higher Education* **16**:460–5.
2. Finch S (1986) *Triad*. Spectra, New York. New edition (2012): Wildside Press, Rockville, Maryland.
3. Wells-Jensen S (2017) *Course Notes*. Bowling Green State University.

4. Uyeno G (2016) Alien interpreters: How linguists would talk to extra-terrestrials. *Scientific American*. Available at: https://www.scientific american.com/article/alien-interpreters-how-linguists-would-talk-to-extraterrestrials. Accessed 2018-04-09.

5. Schirber M (2008) Use grammar to decipher alien tongues. *New Scientist* **200(2678)**:12. doi.org/10.1016/S0262-4079(08)62599-3.

6. Wells-Jensen S (2017) Earth linguistics, xenolinguistics, and the possibility of communication. *NASA Astrobiology Institute, University of Washington*. Availableat:https://nai.nasa.gov/seminars/featured-seminar-channels/university-of-washington-seminars/2017/5/16/earth-linguistics-xenolinguistics-and-the-possibility-of-communication.

7. Porter J, Bonello E and Reynolds F (1998) Effect of epidural fentanyl on neonatal respiration. *Anesthesiology* **89(1)**:79–85.

Chapter

16

The Evolution of Evolutionary Thinking

Abstract

Until recently, experts in evolution, including human evolution, were turned towards the past. They are suddenly invited to look towards the future. Several factors are at the root of the current paradigm shift. As long as the limits of the domination of nature by our species had not been perceived, the concepts of struggle for life survival of the fittest and "selfish genes" were more easily assimilated than concepts such as mutual aid, networking, synergy and symbiosis. Another factor is that modern medicine (particularly reproductive medicine including obstetrics) is neutralising the laws of natural selection, creating inevitable questions about the transformations of our species and the limits of human adaptability. Meanwhile, we are learning from emerging disciplines (such as bacteriology and epigenetics) that have the power to explain how acquired traits can be transmitted to the next generations. Because interpretations are available, it is becoming acceptable to study fast transformations of species induced by changes in lifestyle. Furthermore, since Homo is an eminently social primate, we cannot avoid questions related to the propensity to create working team. These questions lead to consider the evolution of the capacity for empathy, aggressiveness, social intelligence and morality. At the dawn of a new phase in the Lamarckian–Darwinian era, the term "evolution" must recover its original broad meaning, without being exclusively suggestive of one particular mechanism.

Why can evolutionary thinking not easily penetrate the realm of futurology?

Our first interpretation is that creation myths have been, for thousands of years, one of the bases of our cultural conditioning. They imply the view that all species are immutable. Our second interpretation takes into account the new ways of thinking recently induced by Darwinism and Neo-Darwinism. We are now conditioned to associate the evolution of species — including Homo — with the concept of genetic mutation as the ultimate source of variation within populations. This is why time is usually expressed in terms of millions of years among experts in evolution. This is mostly a matter of way of thinking. In reality the terms macroevolution and microevolution have been coined to describe fundamentally identical processes on different time scales. Futurologists, on the other hand, have a tendency to think in terms of decades, centuries, and occasionally millennia. Links are not easy between disciplines that are not familiar with the same units of time.

Learning from Emerging Disciplines

Once more, during the 21st century, we must change our way of thinking. Emerging and fast developing scientific disciplines are explaining how acquired traits can be transmitted to the next generation. Because we now have interpretations at our disposal, it is becoming acceptable to study fast transformations of species induced by changes in lifestyle.

Suddenly, experts in evolution and futurologists have more occasions to share the same units of time. They can communicate. From now on futurologists should not ignore questions about probable transformations of Homo in the foreseeable future. They have reasons, in particular, to focus on the perinatal period, the critical phase of development that has been dramatically modified within recent decades. Until recently, experts in evolution were turned towards the past. They are suddenly invited to look towards the future. We are expecting an evolution in evolutionary thinking.

Among emerging disciplines that explain fast transformations of species, we'll first mention epigenetics. This emerging discipline is based on the concept of gene expression. Some genes may be allocated a kind of label (an "epigenetic marker") that makes them silent without altering the DNA sequences. This marker can be a DNA methylation. DNA methylation, which reduces gene expression, is the best-studied epigenetic marker, mainly because tools have existed to study it. The phenomenon of gene expression is influenced by environmental factors, particularly during "the primal period". We already have a sufficient amount of data at our disposal to claim that, among humans, the perinatal period is a phase of intense epigenetic activity.[1-4] This is a vital issue, since the modes of birth have been radically remodelled during the past decades. Furthermore, it appears today that epigenetic markers (the "epigenome") may be, to a certain extent, transmitted to the following generations. This is why epigenetics is one of the disciplines providing interpretations to fast transformations of species. Transgenerational epigenetic inheritance has been documented for a great diversity of traits in several species. The ability to pass on information about one's environment and one's personal history to descendants could be evolutionary advantageous.[5,6] We cannot help mentioning the premonitions of pioneers such as the followers of Carl Jung, who had introduced the concept of psychogenealogy.

We should not ignore the current limits of the epigenetic perspective. Scientists are still in a preliminary phase in the exploration of long-lasting differences established during the primal period and intergenerational transmissions of the epigenetic markers. We should not ignore, at the same time, some promising aspects of the epigenetic perspective, as a way to study the aging process. This is why we'll find it necessary to introduce the concept of "epigenetic clock".

Bacteriological perspectives offer other promising ways to anticipate fast transformations of human beings. Today, Homo may be presented as an ecosystem with a symbiotic interaction between the trillions of cells that are the products of our genes (the "host") and the hundreds of trillions of microorganisms that make the "microbiome". Let us recall that the "microbiome revolution" is a consequence of technological advances. As long as bacteriologists could only look at microscopes and cultivate microbes on Petri dishes, they could not see the "unseen majority", since the growth conditions of many microbes are unknown. The turning point started when bacteriologists could dramatically expand their horizons thanks to the power of computer processing and new DNA sequencing technologies.

Although microorganisms have been found in the placenta, we can still claim that to be born is to enter the world of microbes. With the use of multiple modes of microbiologic inquiry, an authoritative American study could not identify a "resident microbiota" in placentas delivered at term by pre-labour caesarean sections.[7] It is plausible that some previous studies had not the power to eliminate misleading contamination. It is also possible that there are occasionally such low-abundance and low biomass microbial communities in the placenta that they are not easily detected.[8] We must also keep in mind that periodontal pathogens in placental tissues have been found in association with adverse pregnancy outcomes.[9]

In practice, the important point is to realise that from the first minutes and the first hours following birth, millions of microorganisms start "occupying the territory". According to the well-known bacteriological concept of "the race for the surface", the first microbes that colonise the baby's body become, to a certain extent, the "rulers of the territory". It is also understood that the initial microbiome immediately starts programming the immune system of the child. This is confirmed, for example, by studies of the correlation between Bifidobacterium abundance in early infancy and vaccine response at two years of age.[10]

In such a renewed scientific context, we cannot help analysing and evaluating the drastic changes in birth environment that took place in less than a century. A century ago, as a general rule, women were giving birth among a great diversity of familiar microorganisms. Today it is the opposite. In the particular case of human beings, we must emphasise that microorganisms that are familiar to the mother are also familiar, and therefore friendly, to the neonate, because in our species the haemochorial placenta is highly effective at transferring maternal antibodies (IgG) from the maternal blood stream to the foetal bloodstream. The basic needs of newborn babies must be interpreted in the light of inter-species differences regarding placental structures and functions. In most mammals, which do not receive significant amounts of antibodies through the placenta, the priority is immediate access to colostrum. In our species, the main questions are about the familiarity and the diversity of the bacteriological environment in the birthing place. We must realise the importance of this topic, since it is about health development.

From now on, epidemiologists endowed with evolutionary thinking are in a position to phrase new questions about the prevalence of dysregulations of the immune system in relation to the bacteriological birth environment. Although the concept of dysregulations of the immune system is related to many pathological conditions, the focus might be first on allergic diseases and asthma, and also on autoimmune diseases. The point is to realise that, in the context of the 21st century, there are two kinds of births from bacteriological perspectives: birth at home and birth elsewhere. Until now, epidemiologists have compared hospital births with... hospital births, focusing on extreme situations such as caesarean sections and exposure to antibiotics.

After raising questions about dysregulations of the immune system, let us open a parenthesis to emphasise that, in the near future, the bacteriological perspective will offer a number of other reasons to challenge the dominant doctrines about the place of birth. For example, epidemiologists will have to interpret the current spectacular discrepancies in Bifidobacterium species abundance in the gut microbiome compared to that in historical reports. Fluctuations in the consumption of early colostrum cannot offer valuable interpretations.[11] We must keep in mind the fast evolution of microorganisms. This is a way to explain that microbes that up until now have been classified as commensal hosts can become dangerous nosocomial pathogens. In other words, antibiotic resistance is becoming a major public health issue. The current evolution of several strains of staphylococcus offers typical examples. *Staphylococcus capitis* is becoming more and more involved in neonatal infections.[12] *Staphylococcus epidermidis* used to be a member of the human microbiome, widely present on healthy skin. Today three multidrug-resistant hospital-adapted lineages of this staphylococcus are emerging.[13] Will there come a time when it will appear irrational that human beings are born in buildings originally designed to treat sick people?

Epigenetic and metagenomic bacteriology are the prototypes of emerging disciplines that offer explanations of one of the main particularities of Homo, which is a high degree of "phenotypic plasticity". This new term is appropriate to refer to the capacity to change appearance and physiology in response to environmental factors, particularly during critical phases of development.[14] A high degree of "plasticity" explains that members of our species managed to adapt to places as diverse as equatorial and polar regions.

Modern Lifestyle and Mendelian Inheritance

Although the focus is currently on the transmission of acquired traits from generation to generation, we must not ignore that several aspects of modern lifestyle are dramatically interfering in what we might call Mendelian inheritance. This is the case of reproductive medicine, including obstetrics. One of the indubitable effects of modern obstetrics is to neutralise the laws of natural selection. Before the age of safe caesarean sections and medicalised contraception, women who had many children were those who were giving birth easily. In traditional French villages, a colloquial term was significantly referring to women who had a dozen children (or more). They were classified as "pondeuses d'enfants" (women giving birth like hens laying eggs). Today, the number of children per woman depends on many other factors than the capacity to give birth. Since the way women give birth is to a certain extent determined by genetic factors, statisticians theoretically have the power to predict the phase of history when nearly all human beings will require medical assistance to be born.

Some concrete and precise examples may be useful to illustrate the effects of such a neutralisation of the laws of natural selection.

The issue of breech presentation at term (buttock first or feet first) is typical. Through a huge and authoritative Norwegian study, we can now claim that the main known factors influencing the presentation of the baby at birth are genetic, with maternal or paternal transmission.[15] This piece of knowledge is provided at a time when it is not more dangerous for the baby to be breech born, thanks to easy and safe techniques of caesareans. In such a context it is possible to anticipate a gradual increased prevalence of breech presentation at term. As long as breech presentation at term was comparatively dangerous, the prevalence of this kind of presentation was limited by a threshold in the region of 3%.

It is worth recalling some details about the Norwegian study in order to evaluate its value. The authors used the national birth registry, based on all births in Norway from 1967 to 2004 (2.2 million births). An original and fruitful aspect of the study was the identification of siblings with the same father and different mother and siblings with the same mother and different father. This is how the authors could conclude that having a breech born father or having a breech born mother are situations that equally multiply by more than two the risks of not being born head first.

We'll even dare to add, although many associated factors should be considered, that the tendency towards more breech births at term seems to be already detectable. The proportion of breech births in the Norwegian registry was 2.5% in 1967–76, 3.0% in 1977–86, 3.2% in 1987–96, and 3.5% in 1997–2004.

After choosing the example of breech presentation at term to illustrate the concept of neutralised laws of natural selection, we'll emphasise that there are many other ways to join the growing population of human beings who are dependent on medicine (and health budgets) from the beginning of their life. When considering the great diversity of potentially dangerous births, we realise the magnitude of the topic.

The risks associated with fetomaternal disproportion, a condition in which the foetus is too large relative to the size of the mother, have offered, until recently, a way to interpret the concept of "evolutive bottleneck". From the time when our ancestors separated from the other members of the chimpanzee family until recently (in terms of evolution), there has been a tendency towards an increased foetal head circumference, until the phase of evolution when a too large maternal pelvis would have compromised locomotion. Then limits have been established. The point is that, in the age of safe cae-sarean sections, the "bottleneck" has disappeared. A baby who is too big, compared with the size of the mother, may be born safely without going through the birth canal. Should we expect a return of the tendency towards an increased average head circumference at birth and, finally, an evolution towards an increased average brain volume?[16]

Although we are focusing on reproductive medicine, particularly obstetrics, we must keep in mind other aspects of medicine that will also interfere with Mendelian inheritance. This is leading us to consider, in particular, the issue of "rare diseases". A rare disease affects a small percentage of the population. Most rare diseases are genetic. In terms of public health, it is an important topic because about 7,000 diseases are currently defined as "rare". It is estimated that 300 million people worldwide are living with one of these little-known ailments. With the development of "precision medicine", it is more and more common to try to "repurpose drugs" to treat such conditions. It is therefore plausible that an increased percentage of the affected population will reach the age of reproduction. Will ...."rare" diseases with a strong genetic component become more "frequent"? It is premature to provide simple answers to this question because there will probably be, in the future, more selective interferences in the embryonic period and even in the pre-implantation period.

There are other aspects of modern lifestyle that will undoubtedly interfere with Mendelian inheritance. For example, an increased genetic diversity among humans will be an effect of the emerging global network of fast and cheap transportation associated with easy intercontinental communication through internet and mobile phones. Until now, isolated populations have been inevitably inbred.

Evolving to Control Evolution

Unnatural selection is a comparatively old concept since, as early 1868, Charles Darwin had published "The variation of plants and animals under domestication".[17] It may be presented as an aspect of the domination of nature that started about ten thousand years ago with agriculture and animal husbandry. The objective is the selection of various desired traits. The concept of unnatural selection is easily understood if illustrated through a typical example, such as the case of "doubled-muscled cattle".[18] It is about breeds of cattle carrying mutations responsible for increased number of muscle fibres and reduced fat deposits. The effect is an improved meat tenderness and therefore a greater commercial value. This example is an opportunity to emphasise that facilitating the transmission of traits considered advantageous may be associated with unexpected side effects. In the case of "doubled-muscle cattle", one of the costly side effects is that the enlarged muscles of calves lead to difficult births and high rates of caesarean sections.

From now on, futurologists endowed with a renewed evolutionary thinking cannot ignore new aspects of unnatural selection. They are aware of the implications of prenatal diagnostic testing. They must also be aware of the probable increased use, in the future, of preconception diagnostic testing. It is possible, for example, to detect carriers of recessive diseases. If both members of a couple are healthy, but carriers of a gene responsible for such an inherited disorder, there is one risk out of four that the child will have the disease. Many of such pathological conditions, such as spinal muscular atrophy, are highly invalidating and associated (until now) with a short life expectancy.

Futurologists are also obliged to give a great importance to the advent of technics of genome editing. With tools such as CRISPR, it is possible to create genetically modified mammals and to even edit the germline so that the effects are hereditary. Futurologists must already imagine a time when, in the case of human beings, most technical, financial, philosophical and ethical obstacles have been overcome. There are already reasons to focus on the risks of uncontrollable changes in unexpected zones of the genome in the case of gene editing. There are also reasons to consider the risks that socially advantageous characteristics become concentrated in certain groups or families.

If such a phase of history is reached, the main issue will be about the traits considered desirable. It will depend upon the conditioning of the first human groups that will have access to the editing process. At the present time, it is plausible that a high intellectual quotient would be at the top of the list of preoccupations. Expanding lifespan would also be a highly probable objective. We have already mentioned the complex issue of rare genetic diseases. But futurologists must anticipate plausible radical changes in terms of ways of thinking. Let us imagine a time when the objective of prolonging the survival of humanity by sending members of our species to another galaxy is deemed unrealistic, if not absurd. Then the main questions will be about solutions to prolong the survival of humanity on planet Earth. What kind of Homo will be able to imagine and make realistic such solutions? Since the first and unavoidable answer is "a homo endowed of long-term thinking", we'll create opportunities to focus on this issue.

After recalling that Homo is an eminently social primate, we'll wonder what kind of human beings can make up groups capable of solving vital problems. In other words, the questions will be about the development of the propensity to create effective working teams, keeping in mind that individuals who belong to a working team are supposed to share a common goal. In such a context, we must start by analysing the human traits that can make team work as effective as possible and how these traits develop. Among the factors that promote cooperative and satisfying relationships, we have already mentioned the important issue of the capacity for empathy as a typical "pro-social emotion": team work implies a mode of communication inside the group that is not purely rational and verbal.[19] The propensity to create effective working teams is also an opportunity to raise questions about the nature and the development of "social intelligence", as the ability to understand others so one can get along and cooperate with them. It has been considered a driving force in developing the size of the human brain.[20]

The development of the propensity to create effective working teams also provides an opportunity to present human morality as a product of evolutionary forces that have survival benefits. It is an advantage to restrain selfishness and excessive individualism that could undermine group cohesion. Moral codes are ultimately founded on basic and universal emotional states. There are obvious links between the concept of empathy, that belongs mostly to the framework of emotions, the concept of social intelligence, that belongs mostly to the framework of cognition, and the concept of morality, that cannot be dissociated from the framework of behaviour. In the same way that we have analysed the reasons to be worried about the current demonstrable declining capacity for empathy, we must also raise questions about a probable decline in morality.

The decline in morality is topical, although it cannot be easily evaluated through scientific methods. According to the socio-cultural milieu one considers, it appears that this decline has different facets. Where political and administrative milieus are concerned, the word "corruption" is more commonly used than ever, at such a point that since 1995 "Transparency International" has published every year a "Corruption Perception Index" in a great diversity of countries. At the same time, it is now officially recognised in the most prestigious scientific literature that a great number of modern researchers are corrupted. It is highly significant that the authoritative journal "Nature" has reported this sentence by the environmental engineers Marc Edwards and Siddharta Roy: "If a critical mass of scientists become untrustworthy, a tipping point is possible in which the scientific enterprise itself becomes inherently corrupt and public trust is lost, risking a new dark age with devastating consequences to humanity."[21]

To evaluate the importance of the topic, we must first recall that the sense of what is right and what is wrong is deep-rooted among social mammals in general. In other words, all gregarious mammals adhere to moral codes.[22] This has been widely studied among primates and other mammals such as elephants.[23,24] We have new theoretical reasons to assume that the expression of the moral code is dependent on the oxytocin system, since oxytocin has well demonstrated behavioural effects and may be presented as a hormone involved in sociability. Until recently, human parturition implied an intense activation of this physiological system. Today, in the age of pharmacological substitutes for natural hormones and safe caesarean sections, physiological phenomena are usually neutralised. What is the future of an underused function? Furthermore, because of the high prevalence of induced and augmented labours, the brains of many foetuses, at a critical phase of their development, are now exposed to high concentrations of synthetic oxytocin. The concentration of synthetic oxytocin in the maternal blood stream must be high to be effective, because its release is not pulsatile. If we add that high concentrations of synthetic oxytocin can reach the developing brain after crossing the placenta and the immature foetal blood–brain barrier, we provide an accumulation of reasons to raise questions related to the future of the human oxytocin system.[25]

Can we dream of a time when capacity for empathy, social intelligence and morality become dominant themes among futurists and evolutionists?

Mutual Aid as a Factor of Evolution

From the work of Alfred Wallace and Charles Darwin, it is commonplace to remember the concepts of "survival of the fittest" and competition. The dominant way of thinking has stifled the voices that have presented mutual aid, cooperation and networking as important factors of evolution. Since we are focusing on the evolution of Homo, as an eminently social and teamworking primate, we must give particular attention to this aspect of evolutionary thinking. In his book, published originally in 1900, Peter Kropotkin completed his own observations by presenting an impressive review of available documents focusing on this factor.[26] Kropotkin gave great importance to an address given in 1880 by Professor Kessler, Dean of St. Petersburg University, at a congress of Russian naturalists. Kessler did not deny the struggle for existence, but he was "inclined to think that in the evolution of the organic world — in the progressive modification of organic beings — mutual support among individuals plays a much more important part than their mutual struggle".

Just as Kessler had not denied the struggle for existence, Darwin had also considered cooperation as a factor of evolution, particularly in the case of Homo. In "*The Descent of Man*", he wrote: "The small strength and speed of man...are more than counterbalanced, firstly, by his intellectual powers...and, secondly, by his social qualities which lead him to give and receive aid from his fellow-men. No country in the world abounds in a greater degree with dangerous beasts than Southern Africa; no country presents more fearful physical hardships than the Arctic regions; yet one of the puniest of races, that of the Bushmen, maintains itself in Southern Africa, as do the dwarfed Esquimaux in the Arctic regions." Darwin tacitly reintroduced the concept of "*mutual aid*" in "*Expression of Emotion in Man and Animals*" when documenting such emotions as grief, love and sympathy.

We are not contrasting the writings of Darwin and the writings of others. We are considering how the evolutionary theories have been perceived until now. The point is to observe that, as long as the domination of nature was the basis of our cultural conditioning, the concept of struggle for life, survival of the fittest and "selfish genes" were more easily assimilated than concepts such as mutual aid, cooperation and networking. It is significant that, suddenly, terms such as symbiosis and synergy are emerging key words in evolutionary biology.[27,28]

Today, futurologists who are ready to explore probable transformations of Homo must be guided by a fast "evolution of evolutionary thinking", induced by valuable interpretations of the transmission of acquired traits and the high degree of "phenotypic plasticity" in our species, and also by a renewed focus on long-term thinking and cooperation. At the dawn of a new phase in the Lamarckian–Darwinian era, the term "evolution" must recover its original broad meaning, without being exclusively suggestive of one particular mechanism of the transformations of the species.

References

1. Schlinzig T, Johansson S, Gunnar A, *et al.* (2009) Epigenetic modulation at birth — altered DNA-methylation in white blood cells after Caesarean section. *Acta Paediatr* **98**:1096–9.
2. Almgren M, Schlinzig T, Gomez-Cabrero D, *et al.* (2014) Cesarean delivery and hematopoietic stem cell epigenetics in the newborn infant: implications for future health? *Am J Obstet Gynecol* **211(5)**:502.e1–8. doi: 10.1016/j.ajog.2014.05.014.
3. Godfrey KM, Sheppard A, Gluckman PD, *et al.* (2011) Epigenetic gene promoter methylation at birth is associated with child's later adiposity. *Diabetes* **60(5)**:1528–34. doi: 10.2337/db10-0979.
4. Franz MB, Poterauer M, Elhenicky M, *et al.* (2014) Global and single gene DNA methylation in umbilical cord blood cells after elective caesarean: a pilot study. *Eur J Obstet Gynecol Reprod Biol* **179**:121–4. doi: 10.1016/j.ejogrb.2014.05.038.
5. Lim JP and Brunet A (2013) Bridging the transgenerational gap with epigenetic memory. *Trends Genet* **29(3)**:176–86. doi: 10.1016/j.tig.2012.12.008.
6. Yehuda R and Lehrner A (2018) Intergenerational transmission of trauma effects: putative role of epigenetic mechanisms. *World Psychiatry* **17(3)**:243–57. doi: 10.1002/wps.20568.
7. Theis KR, Romero R, Winters AD, *et al.* (2019) Does the human placenta delivered at term have a microbiota? Results of cultivation, quantitative real-time PCR, 16S rRNA gene sequencing, and metagenomics. *Am J Obstet Bynecol* **220(3)**:267.e1–267.e39. doi. org/10.1016/j.ajog.2018.10.018.
8. Seferovic MD, Pace RM, *et al.* (2019) Visualization of microbes by 16S in situ hybridization in term and preterm placentae without intraamniotic infection. *AM J Obstet Gynecol.* pii: S0002-9378(19)30622-2. doi: 10.1016/j.ajog.2019.04.036. [Epub ahead of print]
9. Fischer LA, Demerath E, *et al.* (2019) Placental colonization with periodontal pathogens: the potential missing link. *Am J Obstet Gynecol.* pii: S0002-9378(19)30614-3. doi: 10.1016/j.ajog.2019.04.029. [Epub ahead of print]

10. Huda MN, Ahmad SM, *et al.* (2019) *Bifidobacterium* Abundance in Early Infancy and Vaccine Response at 2 Years of Age. *Pediatrics* **143(2)**. pii: e20181489. doi: 10.1542/peds.2018-1489

11. Henrick BM, Hutton AA, *et al.* (2018) Elevated Fecal pH Indicates a Profound Change in the Breastfed Infant Gut Microbiome Due to Reduction of *Bifidobacterium* over the Past Century. *mSphere* **3(2)**. pii: e00041-18. doi: 10.1128/mSphere.00041-18. eCollection 2018 Mar-Apr.

12. Carter GP, Ussher JE, Da Silva AG, *et al.* (2018) Genomic analysis of multi-resistant *Staphylococcus capitis* associated with neonatal sepsis. *Antimicrob Agents Chemother* **62(11)**. pii: e00898-18. doi: 10.1128/AAC.00898-18.

13. Lee JYH, Monk IR, Gonçalves da Silva A, *et al.* (2018) Global spread of three multidrug-resistant lineages of Staphylococcus epidermidis. *Nature Microbiol* **3(10)**:1175–85. doi: 10.1038/s41564-018-0230-7.

14. Kelly SA, Panhuis TM and Stoehr AM (2012) Phenotypic plasticity: molecular mechanisms and adaptive significance. *Compr Physiol* **2(2)**:1417–39. doi: 10.1002/cphy.c110008.

15. Nordtveit TI, Melve KK, Albrechtsen S, Skjaerven R (2008) Maternal and paternal contribution to intergenerational recurrence of breech delivery: population based cohort study. *BMJ* **336(7649)**:872–6. doi: 10.1136/bmj.39505.436539.BE.

16. Odent M (2004) Towards a super-brainy homo sapiens? In: *The Caesarean*. Free Association Books, London.

17. Darwin C (1868) The variation of animals and plants under domestication. John Murray, London.

18. McPherron AC and Lee SJ (1997) Double muscling in cattle due to mutations in the myostatin gene. *Proc Natl Acad Sci USA* **94(23)**:12457–61.

19. Konrath SH, O'Brien EH and Hsing C (2011) Changes in dispositional empathy in American college students over time: a meta-analysis. *Pers Soc Psychol Review* **15(2)**:180–98. doi: 10.1177/1088868310377395.

20. Clark EV (1983) Meanings and concepts. In: Flavell JH and Markman EM (eds.) *Handbook of Child Psychology, Vol. 3: Cognitive Development* (pp. 787–840). Hoboken.

21. Edwards MA and Siddhartha R (2017) Academic Research in the 21st Century: Maintaining Scientific Integrity in a Climate of Perverse

Incentives and Hypercompetition. *Environmental Engineering Science.* **34(1)**:51–61. doi: 10.1089/ees.2016.0223.

22. Shapiro P (2006) Moral Agency in Other Animals. *Theor Med Bioeth* **27(4)**:357–73.

23. de Waal F (2006) *Primates and Philosophers: How Morality Evolved.* Princeton University Press.

24. O'Connell C and Jackson D (2016) *The Elephant Scientist* (Scientists in the Field Series). HMH Books.

25. Odent M (2011) The oxytocin system of our great granddaughters. In: *Childbirth in the Age of Plastics.* Pinter & Martin, London.

26. Kropotkin P (1902) *Mutual Aid: A Factor of Evolution.* Will Jonson. ISBN: 978-1497333734.

27. Michel Odent (2016) Symbiosis as the antithesis of Domination. In: *Do We Need Midwives* (Chapter 12). Pinter & Martin., London.

28. Peter Corning (2018) Synergistic Selection. World Scientific.

Chapter 17

The Future of Psychotherapy

Abstract

Psychoanalysis and regressive therapies have reinforced the "know thyself" aphorism. Recent scientific advances, on the other hand, are opening the way to goal-oriented therapies based on the keyword "hope". This chapter provides an opportunity to repetitively conclude that modern human beings are "condemned" to develop and cultivate their prospective way of thinking.

Questions about the future of psychotherapies cannot be separated from questions inspired by emerging branches of medicine, such as immuno-psychiatry.

"A caterpillar who seeks to know himself would never become a butterfly".[1] This assertion expressed by André Gide in 1935 is a turning point in our cultural conditioning. Since the age of Socrates, the aphorism "Know thyself" has been an undisputable component of the dominant way of thinking.

The Future of "Know Thyself"

The paradigm shift induced by André Gide will have practical implications if the importance of recent scientific advances is acknowledged. During the second half of the 20th century, the prototype of health-threatening situations has been investigated and described in easy to summarise terms. We have learned that adverse situations are pathogenic when the subject can neither fight nor fly. Whatever the vocabulary used on the American and European continents, and whatever the details of the animal experiments that were providing answers to a new — although basic — question, it became clear that hopelessness, and therefore hope as its opposite, should become key words in all studies of the genesis of good health and bad health. My book "Primal Health", published in 1986, started with descriptions of the seminal experiments by Martin Seligman, in the USA,[2-6] and Henry Laborit, in Europe.[7,8]

The Future of Goal-Oriented Therapies

In such a cultural and scientific context, there is a need for preliminary questions about the future of psychotherapies in general. Answers to such questions must first take into account the fast development of branches of medicine, such as immuno-psychiatry. Will there be a complementary relationship between psychotherapy and emerging medical specialties? We shall not focus on this question. As social primates endowed with language, human beings need interlocutors. This is one of the reasons why we'll assume that there is a future for psychotherapy.

Although a Beotian concerning this matter, I am inclined to theorise that the main role of a psychotherapist should be based on the health-enhancing effects of developing a prospective way of thinking and the capacity to make projects. The prerequisite to be in a situation of hope is to approach life in a goal-oriented way.

We must realise that the advent of psychotherapies based on keywords such as "goal", "project" and "hope" would be one aspect among others of an expected spectacular paradigm shift. From time immemorial and all over the world there have been kinds of psychotherapists we can refer to by giving a broad meaning to the word "shamanism". As a general rule the "shaman" is endowed of the capacity, whatever the way, to put himself (herself) in a transcendent emotional state. Such an emotional state is contagious and is supposed to have healing effects. The use of hypnosis for therapeutic purposes is also based on induced alterations of states of consciousness with reduced peripheral awareness. Before the term "hypnotism" was coined by the Scottish surgeon James Braid in 1843, Franz Mesmer, during the 18th century, had already tried to interpret this mysterious phenomenon previously called "animal magnetism". In both shamanism and hypnotherapy, the short-term objective is to induce a beneficial crisis through the action of one individual on another one.

There was a turning point in the history of psychotherapy, at the dawn of the 20th century, when Freud started to sit unseen in a corner and when he discarded authoritarian hypnosis. "Free association" became possible. Psychoanalysis was born. The maxim "know thyself" was reinforced. Therapies based on an analysis of the past opened the way to a great diversity of more or less popular regressive therapies such as rebirthing, primal therapy, hypnotic regressive techniques, anatheoresis (reliving past traumas in order to understand and release them), and even past life regression. In the current scientific context, at a time when the intergenerational transmission of acquired traits may be interpreted, there is food for thought in the psychogenealogical approach to therapy. According to specialised practitioners, it is possible and beneficial to conquer seemingly irrational fears and a great diversity of difficulties by discovering and understanding the parallels between one's own life and the life of one's forebears.[9]

Although several kinds of behavioural therapies (based on the idea that unhealthy behaviour can be changed) have discreetly changed the focus during the 20th century, one can claim that the advent of goal-oriented therapies based on the keyword "hope" would appear as one of the components of a necessary new paradigm.

Whatever the topic, we reach the same conclusion, time and time again, that modern human beings are "condemned" to explore the future and to develop and cultivate their prospective way of thinking.

References

1. Gide A (1935) *Les Nouvelles Nourritures*. Gallimard, Paris.
2. Seligman ME (1968) Chronic fear produced by unpredictable electric shock. *J Comp Physiol Psychol* **66(2)**:402–11.
3. Seligman ME, Maier SF and Geer JH (1968) Alleviation of learned helplessness in the dog. *J Abnorm Psychol* **73(3)**:256–62.
4. Seligman ME and Maier SF (1967) Failure to escape traumatic shock. *J Exp Psychol* **74(1)**:1–9.
5. Overmier JB and Seligman ME (1967) Effects of inescapable shock upon subsequent escape and avoidance responding. *J Comp Physiol Psychol* **63(1)**:28–33.
6. Seligman ME and Weiss JM (1980) Coping behaviour: learned helpness physiological change and learned inactivity. *Behav Res Ther* **18**:459–512.
7. Kunz E, Valette N and Laborit H (1974) Role of experience in the mechanism of behavioral inhibition and arterial hypertension following exposure to aversive stimuli without possiblity of flight or fight. *Agressologie* **15(6)**:381–5.
8. Laborit H (1980) *L'inhibition de l'action*. Masson, Paris.
9. Schutzenberger AA (1998) *The Ancestor Syndrome*. Routledge.

Chapter

18 The Future of Abbreviations

Abstract

After evaluating the side effects of overspecialisation, we must wonder how interdisciplinary perspectives can be facilitated. We suggest that language is a possible target in the immediate future. Subcultures have always spoken in codes. Jargon has recently met with a dramatic renewal. Specialists and subcultures have always used ingroup languages that are not understood outside a particular context. Jargon has recently met with a dramatic renewal. We focus on one kind of jargon that has developed at a high speed within the past decades: it is based on the use of abbreviations. After presenting typical examples, we reach the conclusion that the main unanticipated and paradoxical effect of the overuse of this kind of language is to impair communication, reinforcing ingroup–outgroup barriers. We suggest the need for an "anti-abbreviation activism".

We have collected and summarised available data about the short phase of maternal preparation for childbirth as a period of transition before the labour starts. This was a point of departure. One of our ultimate objectives is to evaluate the side effects of overspecialisation. Among these side effects we have mentioned a widespread lack of interest in frontiers between scientific disciplines. We have even suggested that overspecialisation tends to make us blind. In such an unprecedented historical context, we'll multiply the question marks. An example would be: how to facilitate interdisciplinary perspectives?

Is Obscurity the Prerequisite for Credibility?

From a practical point of view, we might first consider the effects of language. Specialists and subcultures have always used ingroup languages that are not understood outside a particular context. Jargon is not new but has recently met with a dramatic renewal. At a time when the need to smash the barriers between scientific disciplines is perceived and even openly recognised, it is becoming urgent to assume that obscurity is not the prerequisite for credibility.

We'll focus on one kind of jargon that has developed at a high speed within the past decades. It is based on the use of abbreviations. Abbreviations have a long history: in classical Greece and Rome, the reduction of words to single letters was common. However, the invasion of daily language by abbreviations did not start until the end of the 20th century. We'll notice that the use of abbreviations and sigla increased in parallel with the development of computer sciences and their tendency to shorten words.

It is easy to illustrate and evaluate the evolution of language in the scientific and medical literature. One effective way is to analyse articles signed by a prolific author during a period of about half a century. As a surgeon, I have always been interested in the prevention of deep vein thrombosis and pulmonary embolism as complications of abdominal surgery. I was convinced that prevention should precede the operation. This is why I have collected many articles co-authored by Vijay Kakkar from the late 1960s until his recent death.

Nearly 50 years ago Vijay Kakkar started to demonstrate the advantages of injecting the anticoagulant heparin on the operating table, before using the scalpel. If we consider a 1969 article he co-authored, it is notable that there were no abbreviations in the abstract while, in the full text, there were only a small number of quasi-inevitable abbreviations, such as X-ray and Hg (for mercury).[1] On the other hand, when reviewing an article Kakkar co-authored at the end of his life, we cannot understand the abstract (and the full text) without first training ourselves to decipher abbreviations such as CAD (coronary artery disease), ACS (acute coronary syndromes), SA (stable angina), PBMC (peripheral blood mononuclear cells).[2] Of course we assume that the readers of such an article understand immediately, without any help, HSP60 proteins, Apo B, T cells, IgM, OR, T helper and Th17 cells.

We have reached such a phase in the history of language — particularly scientific and medical language — that many readers often need time and efforts of attention to decipher the meaning of abbreviations…even when the text is related to topics they are familiar with. When I received an "alert" about "NOACs or DOACs — PHA" in relation to DVT, VTE and PE, I could not easily understand that it was about "Novel Oral Anticoagulants" and "Direct Oral Anticoagulants", although I have followed the history of anticoagulants for half a century. I noticed that PHA starts like Pulmonary Hypertension or Public Health…

In the 1980s, starting from theoretical considerations, I anticipated new generations of studies focusing on the possible long-term consequences of what happens at the beginning of human life.[3] As a first step, I found it relevant to suggest a simplified vocabulary easily understood by as many people as possible, whatever their background. I explained why the keyword I had selected was "primal", an old term (already used by Shakespeare) which means "first in time" and also "first in importance". I referred to the "primal period" as the phase of human development (from conception to the first birthday) when our basic adaptive systems are reaching a high degree of maturity. I referred to "primal health" as a basic state of health reached at the end of the primal period, to "primal health research" as a new branch of epidemiology, etc. At the same time, I started to establish the "Primal Health Research Database" by detecting and collecting in the medical and scientific literature epidemiological studies exploring correlations between what happens during the primal period and what happens later on in life in terms of health and personality traits (www.primalhealthresearch.com).

In spite of such a personal background, I confess that I needed time in the 1990s to decipher the abbreviation FOAD (foetal origin of adult diseases) and, more recently, the abbreviation DOHaD, for developmental origin of health and disease. At a time when health professionals should train themselves to think long term, I wonder how many practitioners, particularly obstetricians and midwives, have their attention immediately attracted by the term DOHaD.

Towards an Anti-Abbreviation Activism

Soon after World War II, the leitmotiv of my professor of philosophy (and other French intellectuals) was the promotion of the global language "Esperanto". We were told that it was a way to foster peace by facilitating the unification of the "planetary village". As teenagers we had difficulties sharing this point of view, as if we felt that a language is like a living creature that cannot be artificially designed. We were much more eager to learn English, which was already on the way to become the international language.

Today English is undoubtedly the "lingua franca". It plays the role of universal language imposed by a dense intercontinental network of air lines, exchanges inside the scientific communities, international business, and international tourism, in particular.

In such a context, while we have at our disposal this lingua franca, we find it useful to express warnings about the overuse of abbreviations. Its main unanticipated and paradoxical side effect is to impair communication. Even if flows of abbreviations are not purposely used to obscure meaning to outsiders, they reinforce ingroup–outgroup barriers, at the very time when it appears urgent to develop interdisciplinary perspectives. It also appears urgent to facilitate communication between experts and the general public. The Academy of Medical Royal Colleges took the historical initiative to advise doctors to use the phrase "twice daily" to explain the dosing of a medicine rather than the Latin abbreviation "bd".

Since we are considering the possible transformations of Homo, as an eminently social primate, we found it relevant to raise questions about the future of empathy and morality. Let us complete with questions about the future of politeness. Documents made of abbreviations should be considered impolite: they imply that "my time is more precious than yours".

References

1. Kakkar VV, Howe CT, Laws JW and Flanc C (1969) Late results of treatment of deep vein thrombosis. *BMJ* **1(5647)**:810–1.
2. Ponnusamy T, Venkatachala SK, Ramaniappa M *et al.* (2018) Inverse association of ApoB and HSP60 antibodies with coronary artery disease in Indian population. *Heart Asia* **10(2)**:e011018. doi: 10.1136/heartasia-2018-011018.
3. Odent M (1986) *Primal Health, A Blueprint for Our Survival.* Century Hutchinson, London.

An Irreversible Conviction

Abstract

Modern humans need to urgently develop their capacity for long-term thinking. After offering reasons for optimism and reasons for pessimism, we raise questions about the nature and the limits of prospective thinking. We eventually try to evaluate the importance of cultural conditioning.

Human beings are suddenly condemned to dramatically develop their long-term thinking. This irreversible conviction is compatible with optimistic considerations.

Reasons for Optimism

The main reasons for optimism are offered by scientists who have already developed and expressed a high degree of prospective thinking. This is the case, for example, of the authors of a 500-year microbial experiment, which started in 2014 and will finish in 2514. Scientists find it useful to evaluate to what extent certain bacteria (*B. subtilis*) are able to tolerate many environmental extremes by transitioning into a dormant state as spores, allowing survival under otherwise unfavourable conditions.[1]

Other reasons for optimism are offered by those whose mission is to react to unprecedented challenging situations, such as the management of nuclear waste. Let us recall that certain radioactive elements, such as plutonium 239, will remain hazardous to living creatures for hundreds of thousands of years. Other radionuclides will remain hazardous for millions of years. Thus, certain kinds of radioactive waste must be isolated from the environment for millennia. Experts endowed with long-term thinking are already offering solutions, such as the use of tunnel boring machines to drill a shaft of about 1,000 metres below the surface where rooms or vaults can be excavated. Our optimistic conclusion is that, in exceptionally challenging situations, human beings become able to express a powerful ability for prospective thinking.

In spite of a renewed degree of awareness, the reasons for optimism are weaker when focusing on issues such as the effects of human activities on climates and the multiple effects of the extensive use of non-biodegradable plastics.

Who Can Study Long-term Thinking?

After considering reasons for optimism, we must once more recall that one of the main reasons for pessimism is a contrast between a widespread interest in the long-term effects of human activities and a lack of interest in the probable fast transformations of Homo. It is as if there is an imbalance between two facets of long-term thinking. How can this imbalance be corrected? It is a Catch-22: only long-term thinking scientists might realise the importance of studying the genesis of…long-term thinking.

Is Prospective Thinking Inherent in Human Nature?

It is certain that, with the recent advent of agriculture, about 10,000 years ago, our ancestors were obliged to reinforce their ability for prospective thinking, at least in terms of season. We already have the proof that, several millennia ago, some post-Neolithic humans had already expressed an extraordinary capacity for prospective thinking. Let us just mention, as a typical example, the case of the Egyptian architect Imhotep, who designed the pyramid of Djoser.

Since we are raising questions about universal aspects of human nature, we must consider the long phases in the history of mankind that preceded the domination of nature through the domestication of plants and animals. It is commonplace to identify our pre-agricultural ancestors as hunter–gatherers who were taking advantage, on a day to day basis, of what nature could offer. We might reach the simplistic conclusion that our Palaeolithic ancestors had no reasons to use and therefore to develop and cultivate their prospective thinking.

We must keep in mind that the way we commonly visualise pre-agricultural Homo is truncated, because palaeontologists, as fossil hunters, can only study human beings who were living inland before the spectacular elevations of sea levels that preceded the Neolithic revolution. They cannot study fossils of humans who have been living in coastal areas for hundreds of thousands of years. They cannot study "Homo navigator". There is no doubt that the Palaeolithic "Homo navigator" had a huge capacity to make projects.

To illustrate the undisputable potential for prospective thinking of pre-agricultural Homo, we'll just recall that our ancestors migrated from Sundaland (which included what we now call Vietnam, Malaysia and Indonesia) to the ancient continent of Sahul (now divided into Australia and New Guinea). The use of appropriate watercraft more than 50,000 years ago is the proof that our ancestors were endowed of the capacity to make and achieve long-term projects. It would have been impossible to design and build overnight the kinds of boats able to carry men and women through a 1,000 km long band of islands and at least 10 ocean straights.

We are in a position to conclude that the ability for long-term thinking is inherent in human nature, but the need to develop this potential can fluctuate according to a great number of historical, geographical and social factors.

How to Select Twenty-First Century Decision-Makers

In the age of overspecialisation, there are obvious individual differences in the need to develop and to use long-term thinking. A gerontologist, as a doctor who is advising people over 80, has few reasons to think long term, compared with a doctor specialised in foetal medicine. Theoretically, we might claim that certain decision-makers, particularly politicians, are those who have developed a high capacity to look towards the far future. In reality it is, more often than not, the opposite. In 1979, in "Genese de l'homme écologique", I ironically analysed the incompatibility between ecological awareness, based on long-term thinking, and political ambition, that leads to focus on short-term challenges.[2] How should we be selecting decision-makers?

In spite of such individual differences regarding the need to use long-term thinking, the way decision-makers are selected should be considered a secondary issue. Decision-makers are human beings: they are part and parcel of our social milieu. At the dawn of a possible paradigm shift, we must first observe and, to a certain extent, we must try to influence the evolution of collective ways of thinking. This is the primary issue. Let us associate the key terms "prospective thinking" and "cultural conditioning".

References

1. Ulrich N, Nagler K, Laue M, et al. (2018) Experimental studies addressing the longevity of Bacillus subtilis spores — The first data from a 500-year experiment. *PLoS One* **13(12)**:e0208425. doi: 10.1371/journal.pone.0208425.
2. Odent M (1979) *Genèse de l'homme écologique*. Epi (Desclée de Brouwer), Paris.

Chapter 20
The Epigenetic Clock

Abstract

In the near future, researchers will have at their disposal a reliable tool to compare chronological age and physiological age. Thanks to "biological clocks" such as those using epigenetic markers or telomere length, it should become possible to explore the possible long-term non-specific effects on health of frequent 21st century interferences in the "primal period". Medicalised conception, ultrasound exposure during embryonic life and foetal life, labour induction, pre-labour caesarean sections, exposure to high concentrations of synthetic oxytocin during the birth process, and multiple vaccinations in early infancy are presented as typical examples of new interferences.

From Gilgamesh to Steve Horvath

Death has always been a major preoccupation among humans, who know that they are mortal. It is significant that, in the earliest surviving great work of literature, Gilgamesh undertook a long and perilous journey to try to discover the secret of eternal life. From time immemorial, there have been countless ways to interfere in the timing and the modalities of death, from suicide to the quest for eternity. Humans have aspired to penetrate the mysteries of the aging process, pushed by the ulterior motive to slow it down and even to reverse it.

Today, in a renewed scientific context, it is commonplace to try to provide new answers to rephrased old questions. In the 1980s, in Germany, three young men with a scientific background had regular meetings to discuss mathematics and scientific topics. They were Steve Horvath, his identical twin Markus, and their friend Jörg Zimmermann. It is significant that they formed the "Gilgamesh project". At their final meeting in 1989, the trio made a solemn pact: to dedicate their careers to pursuing science that could prolong healthy human life.[1] This is how Steve eventually became a human geneticist and biostatistician at the University of California, Los Angeles (UCLA), feeling poised to make good on the promise.

The end of the first decade of the 21st century was a turning point for scientists studying the process of aging. In 2009, Elizabeth Blackburn, Carol Greider and Jack Szostak were awarded the Nobel Prize in Physiology and Medicine. They had discovered that telomeres — protective caps on the ends of chromosomes — shorten with age. For researchers, these findings were suggesting possible ways to contrast chronological age and biological age. At the same time, epigenetics was taking off. This was obviously a turning point in the career of Steve Horvath. As a scientist tied to the "Gilgamesh contract", he immediately understood that the aging process could be looked at in the framework of this new discipline, based on the concept of gene expression. It was technically possible and comparatively easy to evaluate DNA methylation, an "epigenetic marker" that make genes silent without altering the DNA sequences. It was not utopian to study how the speed of the aging process may be influenced by environmental factors and life events. It was realistic to plan the design of "an epigenetic clock".

During the second decade of the 21st century, the history of the epigenetic clock gained momentum. As early as 2011, Steve Horvath's team demonstrated that estimations of the age of a person are possible, based on a biological sample alone: a measurement of relevant sites of the genome could be a tool to predict the risk of age-related diseases and to tailor interventions based on the epigenetic age instead of the chronological age.[2] In 2013, Steve Horvath provided evidence that DNA methylation age measures the cumulative effect of an "epigenetic maintenance system" and that the "epigenetic clock" can be used to address a host of questions in developmental biology, cancer and aging research.[3] In 2015, the same team of researchers revealed that measures of accelerated aging are traits that predict mortality, independently of health status, lifestyle factors, and known genetic factors.[4]

In January 2019, a new step was reached when it was revealed that "DNA methylation GrimAge", as an epigenetic clock based on estimations of plasma protein levels, can strongly predict lifespan and healthspan.[5] Now researchers have at their disposal a biological clock which is impressive with its accuracy and prides new reasons to focus on the concept of timing. Are we entering a new phase in the history of Primal Health Research?

The Future of Primal Health Research

When a tool is available, the first steps are to become aware of its potential functions and to learn how to use it. This is the case of the Primal Health Research Database (primalhealthresearch.com). In the future we'll need to improve the way we take advantage of this collection of epidemiological studies. From a practical perspective, when considering the genesis of a health condition that is not purely genetic, the important point is to have some clues about the critical period for gene–environment interaction. The main questions are expressed in terms of timing. This is exactly the kind of information provided by our database: in the age of overspecialisation, the database has the power to detect unexpected links between diseases.

In such a context, I tested the hypothesis that when two pathological conditions or personality traits share the same critical period for gene–environment interaction, we should expect further similarities, particularly from clinical and pathophysiological perspectives. For example, the keywords "autism" and "anorexia nervosa" (but not bulimia nervosa) lead to studies suggesting that for both conditions the perinatal period is critical. I took this example to look at other possible links between these pathological entities.[6]

From a clinical perspective, several teams have independently emphasised the importance of autistic traits in anorexia nervosa. Deficits in the processing of oxytocin have been demonstrated in both cases. Autistic groups have significantly lower blood oxytocin levels than normal groups, and oxytocin levels increase with age in the normal group only. In autistic groups there is a high ratio of intermediates of oxytocin synthesis (OX-T) to the nonapeptide oxytocin (OT). On the other hand, it has been reported that the level of oxytocin in the cerebrospinal fluid of anorexic women is significantly lower than the level of oxytocin in bulimic and control subjects. Scanning data reveal similar asymmetric functions with left hemisphere preponderance in autistic spectrum disorders and anorexia. Such an accumulation of similarities from a great diversity of perspectives suggests that anorexia nervosa might be considered a female variant of the autistic spectrum. A plausible interpretation is that prenatal exposure to male hormones might protect against the expression of this disease: girls who have a twin brother are at low risk for anorexia nervosa, compared with girls who have a twin sister, and with controls.

This allusion to the links between autism and anorexia nervosa is an opportunity to recall that, in our database, we usually report correlations established by epidemiological perspectives without suggesting interpretations. However, emerging scientific disciplines are now offering such plausible interpretations that the temptation to reduce the gap between correlation and cause and effect relationship is getting strong. For example, a growing body of studies has been recently published, seeking to explain a link between epigenetic modifications and the development of autoimmune disorders such as type 1 diabetes.[7] If we consider that the prevalence of such disorders is increasing, that correlations have been established with the mode of birth, and that there is an intense epigenetic activity in the perinatal period, we cannot help thinking in terms of cause and effect.

Anyway, from now on, one of the priorities will be to explore the long-term non-specific effects on health of invasive and powerful modern ways to interfere in the phase of human development during which the basic adaptive systems are reaching a high degree of maturity. Let us recall, as typical examples of frequent interferences, medicalised conception, labour induction, pre-labour caesarean sections, exposure to high concentrations of synthetic oxytocin during the birth process, and multiple vaccinations in early infancy. Even if prospective randomised trials were ethically acceptable, a long delay would be necessary before getting preliminary results.

It is plausible that, in the near future, other kinds of biological clocks will be tested and eventually become available. For example, researchers might consider recent studies indicating that changes in various histone modifications have a significant influence on the aging process.[8] There are also reasons to take into account that the little known "genomic instability" — the increasing frequency of mutations in our DNA — contributes to aging.

Since health and aging are inseparable topics, we assume that the advent of reliable biological clocks will initiate a new phase in the history of "Primal Health Research". It will help us to rephrase elementary questions about factors accelerating or slowing the aging process and also to re-evaluate the comparative importance of the different phases of primal period.

References

1. Gibbs WW (2014) Biomarkers and ageing: The clock-watcher. *Nature* **508(7495)**:168–70. doi: 10.1038/508168a.
2. Bocklandt S, Lin W, Sehl ME, *et al.* (2011) Epigenetic predictor of age. *PLoS One* **6(6)**:e14821. doi: 10.1371/journal.pone.0014821.

3. Horvath S (2013) DNA methylation age of human tissues and cell types. *Genome Biol.* **14**:3156.
4. Marioni RE, Shah S, McRae AF, *et al*. (2015) DNA methylation age of blood predicts all-cause mortality in later life. *Genome Biol* **16**:25. doi: 10.1186/s13059-015-0584-6.
5. Lu AT, Quach A, Wilson JG, *et al*. (2019) DNA methylation Grim-Age strongly predicts lifespan and healthspan. *Aging (Albany NY)* **11(2)**:303–27. doi: 10.18632/aging.101684.
6. Odent M (2010) Autism and anorexia nervosa: Two facets of the same disease? *Med Hypotheses* **75(1)**:79–81. doi: 10.1016/j.mehy.2010.01.039.
7. Mazzone R, Zwergel C, Artico M, *et al*. (2019) The emerging role of epigenetics in human autoimmune disorders. *Clin Epigenetics* **11**:34. doi.org/10.1186/s13148-019-0632-2.
8. Molina-Serrano D, Kyriakou D and Kirmizis A (2019) Histone modifications as an intersection between diet and longevity. *Front Genet* March 12, 2019. doi.org/10.3389/fgene.2019.00192.

21 The Future of Socialised Birth

Abstract

It is easy to explain that today, where childbirth is concerned, we have reached the limits of the domination of nature. In the age of pharmacological substitutes for natural hormones and safe caesarean sections, only an insignificant number of women, at a global scale, still give birth to babies and placentas thanks to the release of what is now considered a cocktail of hormones of love. Rendering love hormones useless for having babies is a turning point in the history of our species. If the limits of human adaptibility have been reached, the only valuable strategy is to take another direction. After combining what we can learn from physiological perspectives, particularly the concept of reduced self-control as an effect of reduced neocortical activity, what we know about non-socialised childbirth in pre-agricultural societies, and what I have learned as a practitioner, I conclude that it is urgent to challenge thousands of years of cultural conditioning and to consider how and to what extent childbirth can be "desocialised". Can we imagine such a paradigm upheaval so that the need for privacy is recognised? Meanwhile, the development of hypno-suggestive methods in childbirth is justified, even inescapable, as an adaptation to socialised birth.

People my generation are likely to have heard of teenagers who, after concealing or ignoring their pregnancy, just went to the loo and gave birth. After thousands of years of socialised birth, such anecdotes provide food for thought. In all cases the mothers were young. They had snapped their fingers at the rules established by the cultural milieu. They had not read anything about childbirth. Furthermore, the babies were born in complete privacy.

Such stories (outside the related field of "denial of pregnancy") are precious because they are now exceptionally rare. We must keep in mind that the prerequisite for an authentic "unsocialised" birth is weak cultural conditioning. In the context of the 21st century, it still happens occasionally, and often by chance, women are alone when giving birth. However, the power of the conditioning leads us to classify these births as socialised. There are several ways to interpret recent and fast changes in the dominant conditioning. One of them is to keep in mind that the world illiteracy halved during the past 50 years, with a progress towards gender parity. This tendency has been spectacular in parts of the world such as southern Asia and sub-Saharan Africa. The extreme current rarity of unsocialised birth is also related to easy access to modern methods of contraception.

At a critical period in the history of socialised births, we must dare to learn from such anecdotes that were not exceptionally rare until the middle of the 20th century. From a historical perspective, it is easy to explain that today, where childbirth is concerned, we have reached the limits of the domination of nature. In the age of pharmacological substitutes for natural hormones and safe caesarean sections, only an insignificant number of women, at a global scale, still give birth to babies and placentas thanks to the release of what is now considered a cocktail of hormones of love. Rendering love hormones useless for having babies is a turning point in the history of our species. Having reached such limits, the only valuable strategy is to take another direction. Is it possible to "desocialise" childbirth?

To suggest answers to this question, we'll combine two complementary perspectives as a way to improve our knowledge of universal aspects of human nature. We'll offer a synthesis of documents about childbirth in Palaeolithic societies; that is to say among human groups that had not yet domesticated plants, animals and, to a certain extent, members of our own species. At the same time, we'll refer again to the physiological perspective, keeping in mind that it is a way to transcend cultural particularities. We must constantly repeat that today the primary objective should be a better understanding of the physiological processes: *as a first step, it would be dangerous to reduce caesarean section rates.*[1] Then we'll be in a position to refer to labour pain as a central issue for all students of human nature.

Palaeolithic Births

One of the most useful written documents about childbirth in pre-literate and pre-agricultural societies is the book by Daniel Everett "Don't sleep, there are snakes".[2] The author — a male missionary and a linguist — spent nearly 30 years of his life among the Pirahãs, who live in the Amazonian Brazilian jungle by the Maici River. Neither the blurb presenting the book nor the numerous published endorsements mention what Everett wrote about the way women give birth in that ethnic group. It is only in the middle of a chapter titled "Material Culture and the Absence of Rituals" that precious information is incidentally provided.

The Pirahãs have kept many characteristics of Palaeolithic societies, since preparing and planting fields of manioc started during the 20th century. The use of imported machetes is also recent. In such a context, one must read with attention what Daniel Everett wrote about childbirth. A woman usually gives birth by herself, and there is no special place to be in labour. It depends upon the season. In the dry season, when there are beaches along the Maici, a common form of childbirth is for the woman to go alone into the river up to her waist, then squat down and give birth, so that the baby is born directly into the river. Not only is there no concept of a birth attendant but, furthermore, the attraction of labouring women towards water is confirmed as a widespread human behaviour. This is probably the only written document about an ethnic group where babies are occasionally born in water.

There are obvious common points between the report by Daniel Everett and what Marjorie Shostak and her husband Melvin Konner wrote about the "solitary and unaided births" among the African hunters and gatherers !Kung San, who live in the Kalahari desert.[3]

Having spent nearly two years with the !Kung around 1970, Marjorie Shostak, as a woman, became intimate with some local women, particularly Nisa, who gave birth to four babies in the 1930s and 1940s, at a time when the local people were still living as their ancestors had done before them — gathering wild plant foods and hunting wild animals in their semi-arid environment.[4] Although Nisa was aware of a new tendency to socialise the event, she always managed to avoid the presence of other people:

"I have always refused to give birth with anyone there. I have always wanted to go alone. Because, although people try to help you by holding and touching your stomach, they make it hurt more. I did not want them to kill me with any more pain. That's why I always went by myself".

In 1978, at a conference of "ethno-obstetrics" in Gottingen, Germany, I had the opportunity to watch the films by Wulf Schiefen-hövel (from Max Planck Institute) among the Eipos, who live in the highlands of New Guinea. The Eipos were not perfectly representative of a pre-agricultural ethnic group, since they had gardens and pigs. However, they still had Palaeolithic characteristics. The births were not socialised and, in the films made by Wulf and his wife, women are seen giving birth in the bush, without any assistance.

We'll emphasise that these documents are precious pieces of information about lifestyle in Palaeolithic groups living on three different continents. The similarities are striking. They confirm that the socialisation of childbirth started with the Neolithic revolution... not more than 10,000 years ago.

Labour Pain Revisited

The behaviour of Palaeolithic women is in line with the concepts of modern physiology. In a renewed scientific context, we cannot ignore the physiological system of protection against pain. Among humans, a reduction of neocortical activity and the release of substances such as endorphins and oxytocin are undoubtedly essential components of this system. When the neocortex is at rest, peripheral messages are processed differently and they don't have the same lasting effects: there is a depression of memory. The depression of memory has obvious protective effects. It is also an effect of the well-known properties of opiates in general, and therefore of endorphins. Furthermore, the amnesic effects of oxytocin are highly probable: memory tests have been used after a single dose of intranasal oxytocin.[5]

Old questions must be rephrased at a time when it is easy to explain that one cannot artificially extract labour pain and preserve the other links of the chain of physiological events.[6] All components of the physiological analgesic system play multiple roles. For example, beta-endorphins (the main endorphins) are releasers of prolactin, involved in maternal behaviour and milk secretion. We don't need long developments to refer again to the concept of neocortical inhibition and to recall the complex mechanical and behavioural effects of oxytocin.

Once more, the primary question should be: how to protect the physiological processes in the perinatal period against possible inhibitory factors?

Where to Start?

All components of the socialisation of childbirth may be classified today as possible inhibitory factors. Socialised birth went through many phases, with cultural variants, from the advent of midwifery and the most deep-rooted perinatal beliefs and rituals, up to the current masculinisation and medicalisation of the birth environment. We have eventually reached a historical phase when most women cannot give birth and need to be delivered, one way or another, by the medical institution. What is the future of humanity whose babies are born after labour induction, or by caesarean section or, at least, with pharmacological substitutes for natural hormones? There are reasons for concern, even pessimism.

It is urgent to ask how human births can be desocialised.

There are also reasons for hope. The future of Humanity depends on a new awareness. The sudden emergence of a new awareness is unpredictable. The importance of cultural conditioning implies that the way human beings are born is not just a topic for specialised health professionals and pregnant women. Let us use the analogy of anticipated climatic changes in relation to human activities. We have reached such a phase of collective awareness that it is not a topic reserved to climatologists. Everybody is involved. We have not yet reached that stage where birth is concerned. What will take us forward to the next step before it is too late?

As a point of departure, we'll take another look at how language is used to express, transmit and reinforce the current dominant way of thinking. Everybody may have opportunities to talk or write about childbirth. Those who are on the way towards a new awareness have the duty to pay special attention to the vocabulary they use. Let us imagine a journalist reporting an unexpected birth in a supermarket. Instead of focusing, as usual, on the hero who was around by chance and was able to "deliver the baby" and cut the cord, the journalist might start with a headline about a woman "who gave birth" in an unexpected place. The subject of the active verb would be the mother, not the "hero". Let us imagine an activist who wants to promote "natural childbirth". If she is on the way to accepting that giving birth is an involuntary process one can only protect, she will refrain from using the current disempowering vocabulary focusing on the active role of somebody else than mother and baby, the two obligatory actors. She will avoid words such as "helping", "guiding", "controlling", "coaching" (a term implying the need to be guided by an expert), and still more "supporting" (a term implying the need for an energy brought by somebody else).

Since specialised health professionals are those who have a great number of opportunities to talk and write about childbirth, we must consider their vocabulary with a critical mind. Two terms constantly used by obstetricians translate the dominant way of thinking. The labouring woman is commonly called the "patient", a term highly suggestive of a purely passive role. The other commonly used term is "management", which clearly indicates who are the active persons with responsibility. The overuse of the term "management" in the specialised medical literature may appear unsuitable from the point of view of outsiders, particularly when it is paradoxically associated with adjectives suggestive of passivity. Let us mention, for example, studies contrasting labour induction and "expectant management".[7]

The language used in heterogeneous midwifery circles is often different from the dominant language used by specialised doctors. Terms commonly understood by doctors are not always understood by midwives, particularly in some countries, and reverse. For example, obstetricians know about the "Ferguson reflex" while the concept of "foetus ejection reflex" is usually better understood by midwives. How can one interpret such differences? What can we learn from such differences?

Around 1940, when working with anesthetised rabbits, Ferguson had studied uterine contractions induced by vaginal dilation.[8] It was demonstrated afterwards that in the parturient sheep the "Ferguson reflex" is associated with increased blood concentrations of oxytocin and utero-ovarian venous prostaglandins F levels.[9] It was also demonstrated that these responses are blocked by epidural anesthesia.[10] The results of such studies, focusing on vaginal dilation, have immediately attracted the attention of medical circles.

Niles Newton, on the other hand, looked at the effects of environmental factors on the birth of mice. By focusing on the importance of cortical inhibition, even among non-human mammals, she was studying parturition as a chapter of brain physiology.[11] She was using the term "foetus ejection reflex". It is significant that, compared with the work of Ferguson, the studies by Niles Newton have not attracted the attention of obstetrical circles.

In the 1980s, I suggested that an authentic foetus ejection reflex is also possible among humans, but is usually repressed by neocortical activity. With the support of Niles Newton, I wrote that saving this term from oblivion would be a key to facilitating a radically new understanding of the particularities of human parturition.[12,13] I had observed that, in exceptionally rare situations, women can occasionally experience such a reflex, characterised by a birth after a short series of irresistible and powerful contractions without any room for voluntary movements. When a typical reflex occurs, there is an obvious elimination of neocortical control: women seem to be "on another planet", talking nonsense, behaving in a way usually considered unacceptable regarding civilised women, finding themselves in the most unexpected, bizarre, often mammalian bending forward or quadrupedal postures. The reflex does not always start at the same phase of descent of the foetal presenting part.

It is easy to explain why the concept of foetus ejection reflex is not understood after thousands of years of socialisation of childbirth. It is precisely when delivery seems to be imminent that the birth attendant tends to become even more intrusive. The foetus ejection reflex can be preceded by sudden, explosive expression of a fear with a frequent reference to death.[14] Any attempt to reassure with words can interrupt the progress towards the foetus ejection reflex.[15] In the particular context of a preliterate and pre-agricultural society of New Guinea, Wulf Schiefenhövel could discreetly film women giving birth in the bush, without any assistance, through authentic foetus ejection reflexes similar to those some modern women can occasionally experience in ideal situations.[16] In general, any interference tends to bring the labouring woman "back down to Earth" and tends to transform the foetus ejection reflex into a second stage of labour which involves voluntary movements.

Today, there is no simple recipe to overcome thousands of years of cultural conditioning. However, I can describe an environment that is compatible with an authentic foetus ejection reflex, even in the case of highly civilised modern women. The reflex is more likely to occur in a small dark room at a comfortable ambient temperature, with nobody around, apart from one low profile and silent mother figure sitting in a corner.

The popularisation of the concept of foetus ejection reflex, as a consequence of a renewed understanding of birth physiology, would be a critical step towards a certain degree of desocialisation of childbirth. Can we present authentic midwifery as the art of *protecting* an environment compatible with a fetus ejection reflex? Meanwhile, the development of hypno-suggestive methods in childbirth is justified, even inescapable, as an adaptation to socialised birth.[17]

From Adolescence to Menopause

When exploring how human births can be to a certain extent desocialised, so that as many women as possible have babies thanks to the release of love hormones, we have to consider factors other than the birth environment. One of them is the average age at first birth. There is no doubt that, from a physiological perspective, the ideal age for entering motherhood is before 20. To evaluate the current importance of the topic we just need to recall that today, in many countries, a greater number of women have their first baby after the age of 40, rather than before 20. This is a way to explain a dramatic increased dependency on medicine although, occasionally, women over 40 give birth by themselves to their first baby. As a general rule, young women can have surprisingly easy and fast deliveries.

The point is that they are highly vulnerable to environmental factors. Today, their extreme need for privacy is usually overlooked. In other words, it is easy to disturb the birth process in the case of young women. We must also keep in mind some documented negative effects of contraceptive pills before the age of 20, particularly on bone mineralisation.[18]

Can we imagine such a paradigm upheaval that the need for privacy is recognised and that teenage pregnancy is associated with a positive connotation? The ball is in the court of the utopists.

References

1. Odent M (2004) Making sense of rising caesarean section rates: Reducing caesarean section rates should not be the primary objective. *BMJ* **329**:1240. doi.org/10.1136/bmj.329.7476.1240-b.

2. Everett D (2008) *Don't Sleep, There are Snakes*. Profile Books.

3. Eaton SB, Shostak M and Konner M (1988) *The Paleolithic Prescription*. Harper and Row, New York.

4. Shostak M (1990) *Nisa: The Life and Words of a !Kung Woman*. Earthscan, London.

5. Evans SL, Dal Monte O, Noble P and Averbeck BB (2014) Intranasal oxytocin effects on social cognition: A critique. *Brain Res* **1580**: 69–77. doi: 10.1016/j.brainres.2013.11.008.

6. Odent M (2015) In pain thou shalt bring forth children. In: Odent M *Do We Need Midwives?* Pinter & Martin, London.

7. Grobman WA, Rice MM, Reddy UM, *et al.* (2018) Labor induction versus expectant management in low-risk nulliparous women. *N Engl J Med* **379(6)**:513–23. doi: 10.1056/NEJMoa1800566.

8. Ferguson JKW (1941) A study of the motility of the intact uterus at term. *Surg Gynecol Obstet* **73**:359–66.

9. Flint AP, Forsling ML, Mitchell MD and Turnbull AC (1975) Temporal relationship between changes in oxytocin and prostaglandin F levels in response to vaginal distension in the pregnant and puerperal ewe. *J Reprod Fertil* **43(3)**:551–4.

10. Flint AP, Forsling ML and Mitchell MD (1978) Blockade of the Ferguson reflex by lumbar epidural anaesthesia in the parturient sheep: effects on oxytocin secretion and uterine venous prostaglandin F levels. *Horm Metab Res* **10(6)**:545–7.

11. Newton N, Foshee D and Newton M (1966) Experimental inhibition of labor through environmental disturbance. *Obstet Gynecol* **27(3)**: 371–7.

12 . Odent M (1987) The fetus ejection reflex. *Birth* **14**:104–5.

13. Newton N (1987) The fetus ejection reflex revisited. *Birth* **14**:106–8.

14. Odent M (1991) Fear of death during labour. *J Reprod Infant Psych* **9**: 43–7.

15. Odent M (2000) The second stage as a disruption of the fetus ejection reflex. *Midwifery Today* **55**:12.

16. Schiefenhövel W (1978) *Childbirth among the Eipos, New Guinea.* Film presented at the Congress of Ethnomedicine. Gottingen, Germany

17. Odent M. (2019) The future of hypno-suggestive methods in childbirth. *Midwifery Today* **130** (in press).

18. Goshtasebi A, Subotic Brajic T, Scholes D, *et al.* (2019) Adolescent use of combined hormonal contraception and peak bone mineral density accrual: A meta-analysis of international prospective controlled studies. *Clin Endocrinol (Oxf)* **90(4)**:517–524. doi: 10.1111/cen.13932.

Chapter

22 The Evolution of Humanity

Abstract

Before the advent of agriculture and animal husbandry (the "Neolithic crisis"), a human group was a tribe. After that crisis, there have been villages, towns, cities, provinces, states, nations, and international unions. We have suddenly reached an extreme order of magnitude with the concept of "globalisation". From now on, one cannot avoid questions such as: what will happen, in terms of cultural evolution, when (nearly) all human beings are born by caesarean? Can futurologists become evolutionary thinkers? Can evolutionary biologists become futurologists?

Since humans are social primates endowed with the capacity to develop powerful ways to communicate, we must widen the concept of evolution, transcend the individual level, and consider collective traits that might be transmitted to the future generations. We must "adapt" to the continuous and spectacular changes in the meaning of the word "group". Before the recent advent of agriculture and animal husbandry (the "Neolithic crisis"), a human group was a tribe. After that crisis, there have been villages, towns, cities, provinces, states, nations, and international unions. We have suddenly reached an extreme order of magnitude with the concept of "globalisation".

In such an unprecedented situation, we must anticipate a deep paradigm shift.

The recent spectacular steps in the history of childbirth offer an exemplary illustration of the contrast between legitimate short-term and restricted preoccupations and, on the other hand, enlarged ways of thinking. For example, parents should be reassured about the fate of one particular baby born with pharmacological assistance or by caesarean section, because the cultural milieus can compensate many individual deprivations. From now on, the focal questions should be about the evolution of humanity. For example: what will happen, in terms of cultural evolution, when (nearly) all human beings are born by caesarean?[1]

Most of the questions we are raising are associated with obvious reasons for pessimism.

Will there be reasons for optimism on the day when evolutionary biologists explore the future?

Reference

1.   Odent M (2009) Wie steht es um die Zukunft einer durch Kaiserschnitt entbundenen Zivilisation? In: Stark M, *Der Kaiserschnitt*. Elsevier/ Urban & Fischer, Munich.

Index

Printed in the United States
By Bookmasters